Women Changing Therapy

**New Assessments, Values and Strategies
in Feminist Therapy**

Women Changing Therapy

New Assessments, Values and Strategies In Feminist Therapy

Edited by

Joan Hamerman Robbins
Rachel Josefowitz Siegel

Women Changing Therapy: New Assessments, Values and Strategies in Feminist Therapy was originally published in 1983 by The Haworth Press. It has also been published as *Women & Therapy*, Volume 2, Numbers 2/3, Summer/Fall 1983.

Harrington Park Press
New York • London

ISBN 0-918393-07-8

Published by

Harrington Park Press, Inc.
12 West 32 Street
New York, New York 10001

EUROSPAN/Harrington
3 Henrietta Street
London WC2E 8LU England

Harrington Park Press, Inc., is a subsidiary of The Haworth Press, Inc., 12 West 32 Street, New York, New York 10001.

Women Changing Therapy: New Assessments, Values and Strategies in Feminist Therapy was originally published in 1983 by The Haworth Press, Inc. It has also been published as *Women & Therapy*, Volume 2, Numbers 2/3, Summer/Fall 1983.

Library of Congress Cataloging in Publication Data

Main entry under title:

Women changing therapy.

    Reprint. Originally published: New York : Haworth Press, c1983.
    "Has also been published as Women & therapy, volume 2, numbers 2/3, summer/fall 1983"—T.p. verso.
    Includes bibliographies.
    1. Feminist therapy. 2. Women—Mental health.
I. Robbins, Joan Hamerman. II. Siegel, Rachel Josefowitz.
RC489.F45W65   1986   616.89'14'088042   84-19276
ISBN 0-918393-07-8 (pbk.)

In memory of my mother
Frieda Shur Josefowitz

and

for my daughter Rebecca Robbins
who continues to grapple with the
expanded possibilities that are
now a woman's life.

CONTENTS

Foreword

Women are changing, the world is changing and women are changing the world. What a challenging time to be living on this planet! Two women, Joan Hamerman Robbins and Rachel Josefowitz Siegel, have taken on the challenge of organizing a book on feminist therapy out of their own and others' participation in the Women's Institutes of the American Orthopsychiatric Association. This is a daring book, one which offers new understandings and techniques for changing our lives—as therapists and clients—through the feminist therapy process.

More women are writing these days and are ready to share their insights with a larger audience. In *Women & Therapy,* A Feminist Quarterly and in *Women Changing Therapy* we are presenting articles written by authors who are being published for the first time. The timing is right. The need is here: to redefine what the therapy process is all about from a feminist perspective. And women are willing to take the risk of sharing in print what they know to be of value. *Women Changing Therapy* demonstrates how women are speaking out with potency, clarity, and fresh insights.

Betts Collett
Founding Editor
Women & Therapy
A Feminist Quarterly

Preface

This book is about feminist therapy, about women defining themselves and their own experiences within an egalitarian therapy relationship. It is about women changing society, expanding their horizons and activities, making choices they never made before, and using therapy to facilitate this process. It is a book written by therapists and counselors about innovations and alterations in the theory and practice of therapy, growing out of an expanded awareness, and appreciation of women's perceptions of the world.

This book is about women, clients and therapists, rejecting male-centered definitions, taking off male-colored glasses, and learning to tolerate the confusion and ambiguities of trying out new lenses, finding new perspectives, seeing the world, themselves, each other from different angles. Alice Walker has written: ''. . . you have to git man off your eyeball, before you can see anything a'tall.''* When the world is no longer polarized into rigid definitions of male/female, dominant/subordinate, normal/deviant, new thinking emerges; we can move forward to a fuller integration of knowledge and experience about people.

It is both exhilarating and painful to engage in the process of self-discovery, questioning old assumptions, telling the truth as we experience it. In therapy we learn to tolerate the anxiety and discomfort that are the by-products of such a search. You, the reader, may go through a similar process as you make contact with the disquieting content of these pages. You may respond with enthusiasm to the discovery of truths that validate your own perceptions. Or you may get caught up in feelings of confusion, anger, ambivalence and pain. Upon reflection, we hope you too will find positive and constructive new solutions, new tools and concepts that have specific meaning for you in your personal and professional life.

The making of this book illustrates the kind of supportive and collaborative relationships between women which are at the root of the women's movement, and that enable individual women to stretch their capacities beyond the limits of their early training. The friend-

---

*A. Walker, *The color purple*. New York: Harcourt Brace Jovanovich, 1982.

xv

ships which have grown out of this enterprise have profoundly affected our lives, producing the kind of changes we write about in the book, changes in our selves, in our interactions with the world, and in our ways of doing and understanding therapy.

We, Joan and Rachel, first met in San Francisco, at the 1978 American Orthopsychiatric Association's Institute on Women which had been organized by Jean Baker Miller. We were both drawn to the Institute by reading Jean's book, *Toward a new psychology of women* (1976); it had begun to reverberate within us and in our clinical work. Through her book and her initiative in creating womens' networks, Jean had become a central figure in the development of new ideas about women. The authors and editors of this book are connected to each other through her work and through the Ortho Women's Institutes which she continued to co-organize and inspire. The Institutes became a forum for our interactions, the annual opportunity to present our ideas, clarify and exchange our views, and experience an intellectual and emotional environment that challenged and supported our individual and collective creativity.

In 1979 we met again as members of the newly formed planning collective for the Institute. We got to know each other and to respect each other's work and opinions. The idea of a book was proposed very tentatively at a planning collective meeting following the 1980 Institute in Toronto. Rachel had the dream: a book of the collected papers presented at the Women's Institutes. Joan responded to the dream. Each of us is in private practice and occasionally feels isolated in our own community. The fact that we live 3,000 miles apart added challenge, and maybe a bit of safety to a collaboration that was to become a major and central involvement in each of our lives.

We began with a deep appreciation of the papers that were being presented. We also shared a commitment to the feminist process of paying attention to the quality of our interactions with one another and with our authors, as well as to the end product of our work. Working together on the book since then has cemented a friendship and alliance which empowered us both and without which the project would have been dropped long ago. It has also led us both to do much thinking and talking about the creative potential in women's friendships and support networks.

In the tradition of the Institutes we felt it was important for this book to combine the work of unpublished authors with that of more experienced writers and practitioners. Our selections grew to include authors who presented at more recent Institutes. The papers reflect a commitment to more than one style of exploring knowledge and communicating with each other; we express ourselves in theoretical, clinical and personal styles. Our book is the story of women empowering themselves and each other to think creatively, to express and expose themselves in writing, to learn through trial and error and to act in their own behalf.

Many people, friends, family, clients and colleagues have helped us directly and indirectly in this process and we wish to thank them all, especially for continuing to believe in us and in our project during those moments when we felt most doubtful and discouraged. We also thank our authors for trusting us, correcting us and hanging in there with us; and Betts Collett, editor of *Women & Therapy,* whose input was invaluable during the final phase of the work.

Rachel Josefowitz Siegel
Ithaca, New York

Joan Hamerman Robbins
San Francisco, California

Women Changing Therapy

New Assessments, Values and Strategies
in Feminist Therapy

WOMEN'S ISSUES: NEW ASSESSMENTS

It is the conflict between past and present that makes the stuff of therapy. In this section the authors focus on the conflict between women's early training to become childlike, helpless, submissive, dutiful and devalued daughters, wives, and mothers, and our present hopes and expectations to be self-sufficient, autonomous, fully functioning, valued adult members of society. Jean Baker Miller identifies conflict as the necessary condition that is central to the process of change toward wholeness and equality.

The oppression of women in our culture has taken its toll on female development; stereotyped roles and expectations have kept us from realizing our potential and continue to reinforce a power imbalance between women and men. The denial of our subordination has kept women divided from each other. Paula Caplan delves into the ramifications of such divisions at work and in politics. We blame one another and we blame our mothers for the legacy of restrictions imposed by the patriarchy. Joan Hamerman Robbins traces the sources of such blame back to early family interactions and mother's devalued place in the child's world.

It is not easy to move forward from this place. Our authors acknowledge the complexity of the issues, the internal and external forces that oppose change, and the need to value and appreciate the struggle itself and the gains already made within the context of these difficulties. Recognizing society's mixed message to women, Jessica Heriot observes a range of responses that keep women separated from their own sense of wholeness and wellbeing. She outlines the steps that lead to healing this split.

Conflict and anger which women have been taught to deny and to repress, need to be recognized and harnessed effectively in the process of growth and change. This issue, and its importance in the

1

therapeutic encounter are highlighted by Alexandra Kaplan and her co-authors. The last two papers specifically address women's issues in the larger world: the world of work and of political realities.

The pressures encountered at work are new and unfamiliar to clients and therapists. Women are succeeding as pioneers in occupations that have until recently excluded them. Beth Milwid explores the stresses and sacrifices that confront women competing in workplaces designed by men. Marjorie Braude looks at the consequences of limiting our rights to reproductive freedom. These rights continue to be challenged by church and state; male dominated society continues to assert its ownership of womens' bodies. We need to change these conditions of our oppression using conflict and anger to that constructive purpose.

We are beginning to reject our legacy of weakness and embrace instead our heritage of "energy and richness." We are encouraged by Jean Baker Miller's observation that women are the people most likely to push for a society that is more responsive to individual needs and values, because women understand so deeply and fully what it means to be excluded and oppressed.

The Necessity of Conflict

Jean Baker Miller

Today it is especially women who are putting forward a vision of wholeness. There are deep reasons why women are the people who want to and who can create that vision. And yet—seemingly paradoxically—it is also women who can perceive most clearly and profoundly that we must embrace conflict, claim conflict as our own. An odd-sounding statement perhaps—for we tend to think "who wants conflict?" Indeed, we have all been taught to dread it, hate it, twist ourselves into pretending that it doesn't exist.

This, I believe, is one of the deepest and worst distortions systematically inflicted on us. It is not that we should want to feel torn or in pain, but instead that the search to understand and clarify our own inner conflict can lead to a reduction of anguish and even a transformation of pain into possibilities. To do this, however, I think that we must continue to re-examine the origin and meanings of conflict. In doing so, we can take hold of a key force in our struggle to understand and change ourselves and the world. We already have within us a strong and valid basis by virtue of being women. We have all lived with external and internal conflict from the moment we were born, probably unjustifiably condemning ourselves for it in each instance. To illuminate and embrace conflict, we have to see it as a factor which is present in all of life, but most crucially in women's lives. Indeed, we women have within us the basis for being the quintessential "experts" on conflict. In using our expertise, we can illuminate not only ourselves but the world.

A brief example from one woman's life may make some of these points a bit clearer. S. L. is an aide in a service agency, who is very good at working with clients. She is good precisely because she has incorporated some of the human necessities which have been delegated to women in our society (and also simultaneously kept de-

The author is Director, Stone Center for Developmental Services and Studies, Wellesley College, and Clinical Professor of Psychiatry, Boston University School of Medicine, Boston, Massachusetts.

valued and hidden). That is, she approaches her clients with an attempt to understand them, to be responsive to them, to feel *with* them rather than *above* them and to truly work together with them for their good. Yet, there are times when S. L. becomes apathetic, depressed, doesn't seem to care about her work, and feels a loss of interest in it. Current conditions can depress and discourage anyone, but there were additional factors operating for S. L. For, like many of us, she wanted to find a way to deal with the surrounding destructive milieu. She didn't want to go around depressed but wanted to feel alive and effective. After difficult and often anguishing exploration, she unearthed some clues. One striking discovery was that her depression and immobility began when she especially wanted to *do something,* i.e., when she saw what was wrong in the situation and saw ways to act on it that would be effective—but then felt blocked from acting. She was blocked on several levels. On one level there were the sheer external conditions of the hierarchical structure of her agency. S. L., in low rank, is not given the right nor the power to question, criticize or suggest to those in authority over her. In this S. L. is, of course, similar to most women workers who fill the bottom levels of the hierarchy ordered and structured by those at the top who are men (administrators, in this instance).

This clear external structure has, however, its internal counterpart, which has become self-enforcing for many women, in a much more complex and hidden way. This internalized structure was more difficult to get at. S. L. discovered that at the precise point when she, herself, starts to perceive, criticize or has an idea of how something could be done—and most important, when she sees that she could truly play a role in doing it, an immediate counter-reaction sets in. It's a complicated reaction. It includes fear, and then a feeling that she is bad, evil. This is followed by self-condemnation and self-blame. With it all there is anger, complicated anger. It is anger at the initial event and, also, at the internal entrapped feeling, at the encased way she feels. But S. L. turns this anger into further self-disparagement. To top it off, S. L. at this time is not so good at her work or in the way she acts toward other people. So doesn't this all prove that the self-blame is accurate—she's no good anyhow?

A crucial factor here is that this series of internal events turns on in a flash, the instant S. L. begins her own self-initiated thoughts or actions. These reactions have become so automatic and so complex that they have become very difficult to unravel. (Merely telling S. L. that she should be assertive is not enough—she knows that, but she's depressed and, furthermore, her self-disparagement makes her think she has nothing valid to assert.)

Once unraveled, however, this sequence makes a great deal of sense. In addition, it illuminates women's general situation. The very first step, that is the very first impulse to act out of one's self, has been prohibited for women. This is not what women were supposed to do. Women were defined as being there to serve the needs of others as defined by a male-structured culture. Therefore, the very basic premise that a woman should act—move—out of her own perceptions and motivations has not been a premise that existed in most cultures. This is a very real and very profound factor which still affects most women.

Almost from the moment of birth, there has been instilled in us the inner notion that acting out of one's self is a dangerous, frightening and evil thing. Although such actions are highly encouraged in men, and become very enhancing to men's sense of self, self-worth and self-esteem—they have the reverse effect for many women: threatening one's sense of self and producing a sense of unworthiness, evil, danger—or, at the very least, a sense of conflict and unease. This is a more complex inner threat to add to the clear external threats that punish girls' and women's forthright action. This built-in threat has been a powerful force preventing most women from being able to connect freely with the first basic element of being alive—acting out of one's self and one's desires as one sees them at each moment. It then prevents us from being able to formulate, to know, and state our desires.

Thus, most women have yet to fully tap into all of the energy, power, action, perception, and sense of freedom that comes with a sense "that it is right and good that I do this elemental thing." Instead, we see that acting out of our own perception and motivation becomes a very complex process. The road to recapturing the basic right to see and to do is filled with doubts, questions and often very deep anguish.

Indeed, the whole construction of the world as it has been is one in which only men are the actors. The ways which we have been given to feel, perceive, think; our structure of conscious and unconscious symbolizing; our system of expression—language itself—all have been formulated in terms of this basic construction of the world. They have all been ordered and constructed out of a milieu, a culture which has been centered around the male as actor, sole judge of actions, maker of symbols and language. The male has made himself the location of all power and value. Only such actions as the male culture calls forth are permissible for women. The very experience of having the desire to act, to initiate which all people do have—that very impetus, then, is something which is, in a deep sense, inconceivable. It is in a realm filled with dread—and awe. By contrast, actions which women can conceive of as called forth by others and done for others, actions which a male structure says are right, can often seem easy to do.

It is important to recognize how thorough this structuring has been. If we recognize this, we may be less discouraged at the difficulty, the length, and the depth of the inner conflict that we encounter. Indeed, given the heavy barriers both externally and internally, we can celebrate the many accomplishments that women have already made by establishing that very first premise—the premise that we have the right, the obvious ability and, moreover, the *need* to see and act out of the energy and richness of ourselves.

When we recognize, as we now do, the fact that one half of the human race has been held in subordination to the other half, we see immediately the inevitable conditions for conflict. Nobody, I believe, accepts this kind of subordination. And, of course, a dominant group always makes it look as if there were no reason for conflict; that "the way things are" is right and good. Thus, any girl or woman who feels either an impulse to initiate action or feels an impulse to react against this total constraint inevitably has to feel in conflict with the way things are. Sensing it, women also feel that this perception of conflict must be squelched. The squelching takes forms that have become very subtly systematically woven into the woman's inner psychology; they can be deceptive. A most basic factor here, then, is the factor that the moment most women felt this conflict, we also felt a powerful inner voice saying "if you feel any conflict you must be wrong." Not only are you wrong, you must be somehow bad for feeling it, and in addition, in modern terms, maladjusted, neurotic, sick.

It follows that male-ordered society has been inevitably a very skewed society since it has been led by a group which believes it has to keep half of the human beings in a subordinate position—whether any individual man chooses to do so or not. This group has not been able to encompass many essential parts of life. It could not encompass, for example, full emotional relatedness, mutuality, true empathy, sharing of power, cooperation or creativity because these parts of the human potential would disrupt a structure of dominance.

Since at least some portion of these many parts of life are essential in order for any society to exist at all, the dominant group has sought to have them supplied—by women. Thus, despite all of the suppression, women have "filled in" these key parts of life—mainly within the family, but often in other settings as well. Simultaneously, these aspects have been devalued. For example, although women in general have a much greater sense of the importance of a feeling of connection to other people, this sense of connection with others has not been given its full value in the dominant culture. Instead, it has been disparaged and this situation has led to women disparaging themselves for feeling its importance—for feeling that they want and need these connections. "Why do I seem to need other people?" many women say. "Doesn't it show I really am weak and dependent?" There are many parts of life which have been delegated to woman; or in the dominant culture's terms, relegated to women. Some recent writings are now re-examining and redefining the nature of the characteristics which women tend to develop (e.g., Miller, 1976, 1982; Gilligan, 1982).

Given the heavy weight of all of these factors, I think that we can see the need to take on the fuller exploration of conflict within ourselves and with the dominant culture; and use this exploration for our benefit. We might start by considering some of the following steps: first, stop condemning ourselves for all of the conflict we feel. Second, see that many of the things we have felt have indeed come from conflict but that we have suppressed that conflict. We have tried to twist ourselves and thereby experienced that conflict in disguised forms, such as apathy, depression, phobias, inadequacy, helplessness, and a whole array of other feelings—all making us feel that we really couldn't do anything. Third, we can see that looking at, and understanding conflict can be a key step in illuminating the truth about ourselves and the world. We can then come to see things in a much different way.

Women have developed extremely valuable strengths—some of which I've suggested briefly. The question arises how these strengths have possibly developed in this oppressive situation. I think the answer lies in those parts of life which women have had to furnish for male-dominant society. They are those very parts that are closest to making us full and whole human beings. It is here that the paradox of wholeness and conflict come together. Just because women have "filled in" these parts of life, women are also closer to seeing and feeling wholeness. Further, because women have been in the oppressed position, we are more able to perceive the deficiencies in male-dominant aspirations and are aware of how those aspirations lead away from wholeness. Women, for example, have known how empty and cruel it is to be acted upon by another, rather than having the possibility of *acting with* another.

It then becomes apparent that women can be the people who can most clearly perceive the path toward a concept of wholeness. Women can feel less compelled to adhere to a narrow lifestyle and can be less constrained by the blinders to which those in the position of oppressor must cling. It is also true that women cannot aspire to wholeness without simultaneously recognizing the conflict-producing condition within which we have lived so far. We all reflect this in various ways, and it is impossible to leap over this conflict and its legacy. We cannot expect an instant sense of wholeness. We can, however, search for wholeness while we continue to unearth these conflicts and their sources. As we do that, because we are women, we will find that we inevitably see new things and bring new ways. This is a huge task. We will find ourselves thinking in new terms, even seeking new words because the very way in which experience has been conceived and expressed comes out of a culture which has misconceived and misexpressed much of life.

I have talked about the conflict which must occur whenever one group seeks to use another whole group for its purposes—and certainly when each group is one half of the human race. I've suggested that this external conflict produces an ensuing internal conflict which then becomes elaborated at the psychological level. It's influences shape both basic psychological development and the relationships between people at every life phase. However, I believe that another form of conflict is inherent in all of life. We can think of conflict as a process between that which is beginning or new, and that which is old, or from which we are moving on. This is to say that as everyone grows, there is conflict. This conflict has been made difficult to perceive because we have been living within a structure which seeks to suppress all conflict in order to maintain a *status quo.* Such a structure has kept us from awareness of this most basic conflict, because it has to keep down all conflict. Each person, as she or he grows, is constantly in struggle with the *status quo,* both the *status quo* of her/his current psychological forces and that of the surrounding interpersonal and cultural milieu. She/he is carrying within herself/himself the seeds of an emergent new way of being which will change both herself/himself as well as the external situation. This interaction which each individual brings to the social structure is the inevitable source of life and growth for the whole social unit. Only when we are able to move out of a structure which has been oppressive, will this conflict be able to come forward in its fullness. Then our society can become a continually renewing and changing structure.

Thus, in a sense, women have a double conflict. We are engaged first of all in the huge confict with a structure which is oppressive. At the same time, we are illuminating a future encompassing the conflict of growth.

Women seeking to understand ourselves, illuminate not only ourselves but the forces for growth that patriarchal society has kept undeveloped and hidden from all.

REFERENCES

Gilligan, C. *In a Different Voice: Women's Conception of Self and Morality.* Cambridge, Massachusetts: Harvard University Press, 1982.

Miller, J. B. *Toward a New Psychology of Women.* Boston: Beacon Press, 1976.

_____. Women and Power, *Work in Progress.* Wellesley, Massachusetts: Stone Center Working Papers Series, 1982.

The Double Bind: Healing the Split

Jessica Heriot

THE DOUBLE BIND: HOW IT WORKS

The concept of the double bind is a familiar one. Gregory Bateson and R. D. Laing (1961), looking at the communication patterns of families of schizophrenics, noticed that the double bind characterized the way many families related to each other and to their schizophrenic member. They theorized that a person who is constantly faced with choosing between two "no win" alternatives can become schizophrenic.

> One person conveys to the other that he should do something, and at the same time conveys on another level that he should not, or that he should do something else incompatible with it. The situation is sealed off for the victim by a further injunction forbidding him to get out of the situation, or to dissolve it by commenting on it. The victim is thus in an untenable position. He cannot make a move without catastrophe (Laing, 1969, p 127).

What Bateson and his associates did not realize is that a whole society can "double-bind" a whole group of people. I refer here to the situation of women in our society. To understand how society has double-binded the female half of the population, I have expanded this definition and substituted the specific double messages that society gives to women.

> Society conveys to women that they should find their greatest happiness and fulfillment in giving to, and serving others, and

---

The author is a Social Worker and a feminist therapist. She is a founding member of the Women's Growth Center in Baltimore.

11

at the same time conveys on another level that they are not really valuable for doing this, or that they should be more like men. The situation is sealed off for women by a further injunction that women are abnormal if they do not want to fulfill their role, forbidding them to get out of the situation or to dissolve it by commenting on it. Women are thus in an untenable position. They cannot make a move without catastrophe.

The empirical evidence for the assertion that women are in a societally contrived double bind situation emerged from a now classic study by Broverman, Broverman, et al (1970). In this study male and female clinicians were asked to describe a "mature, healthy, socially competent" man, woman, and adult, by using a check list of male/female personality characteristics. The results of the study made explicit what many women already intuitively knew. A "mature, healthy, socially competent" male person possessed some of the following traits. He was "aggressive, independent, objective, not easily influenced, active, logical, worldly, adventurous, self-confident, and able to separate feelings from ideas." However, a "mature, healthy, socially competent" woman was something other than that. According to the clinicians, a healthy woman was "easily influenced, submissive, passive, illogical, sneaky, dependent, not adventurous, and unable to separate feelings from ideas." *To be a healthy woman by society's standards is to be a sick adult. On the other hand, for a woman to aspire to a societal definition of adulthood is to do so at the cost of her womanhood.*

In our society, women's aspirations to full adulthood have been labelled "abnormal" or "sick." Even today, a woman striving to develop and integrate adult behaviors does so in the face of powerful internal and societal injunctions against violating traditional female roles and male prerogatives. Clearly women are caught in a no-win predicament, where femaleness is devalued and access to adult/male behavior is fraught with conflict. To opt for the traditional female role (with all its accompanying personality traits and behaviors) is to experience oneself to some degree as an inadequate adult: an inferior human being. To opt for the valued adult/male role (with its accompanying personality traits and behaviors) is to violate society's definition of a "normal" woman and to experience feelings that range from a gnawing sense of dissonance to panic.

Looking more carefully at the female role of this no-win bind, we see that typical female personality characteristics fall into two categories: "positive" female traits and "negative" female traits. The first category includes characteristics which are considered valuable and positive *but only for women*. They are considered strange or negative when they occur in men. Some of these traits are: intuitiveness, gentleness, sensitivity, empathy, warmth, sweetness, softness, subjectivity, tenderness, and the ability to be openly loving and caring. Highly prized in women, these qualities are devalued when compared with characteristics commonly associated with adult males. This is because these "positive" female qualities grow out of women's traditional role as nurturer and caretaker; and our society does not value doing and caring for others as much as doing and caring for oneself, which is the socialized goal or mission of men's lives.

The second category, "negative" female traits, includes those which women are seen to possess by virtue of their femaleness but which are viewed as negative for both women and men, such as emotionality, submissiveness, passivity, fearfulness, weakness, vulnerability, helplessness, dependency, irrationality, and childishness. Though these traits are ascribed to the "weaker sex," women do not have a corner on these feelings. As Jean Baker Miller (1976) states, "women have become the carriers for society of certain aspects of the total human experience. The result of such a process is to keep men from fully integrating these areas into their own lives." It has been easier for men to denigrate women as possessors of the frightening and unacceptable feelings of vulnerability, powerlessness, and the need for connectedness than to deal with these feelings in themselves. Women, designated as the natural repositories of these negative feeling states, come to feel like defective models and somehow must deal with this sense of themselves as inferior within the total context of their femaleness.

In identifying with the female pole of the no-win split, women are not rewarded for their devalued "positive" qualities and are punished for their ascribed "negative" qualities. On the other hand, to identify with valued adult/male behaviors and personality traits is to precipitate an identity crisis, evoking feelings ranging from discomfort to fear. The consequences of either choice are untenable.

Women's responses to the double bind form a continuum. On one end are "female identified" women who live out the traditional female role (with its constellation of traits and behaviors) and often suffer the symptoms that we have come to associate with it: low self-esteem, excessive dependency, anxiety, and fearfulness. At the other end of the spectrum is a much smaller group of women, "male identified," who act out the traditional adult/male role. In exchange for their adult status, they cut themselves off from their sense of femaleness. At the mid point of the continuum are women who feel split between their desire to be valued as effective adults and their need to be seen as acceptable women. They walk a tight-rope between adulthood and womanhood. They are caught in the double bind which requires them to choose between two untenable alternatives. As a result, their lives are fraught with ambivalence, anxiety, contradictions, and confusion.

A woman's adaptation to the double bind affects her life choices, relationships and work. Each mode of adaptation generates psychological problems and deprives a woman of access to her full potential. Each adaptation also provides the opportunity to develop qualities, skills and behaviors that are positive, valuable, and useful.

Every woman finds her own way to cope with the double bind split. She is influenced by the values of her family of origin, the role models her mother and father presented, and the events in her life that brought home messages about what and who women should be.

YOU CAN'T WIN FOR LOSING: THREE ADAPTATIONS TO THE NO-WIN SPLIT

The "Female Identified" Woman

The strongest and clearest message that women have received, and to a large degree still receive, is that they should find their greatest happiness and fulfillment in living for and through others; specifically husbands and children. We know this group of women well. They flood the offices of private therapists, mental health clinics, and psychiatric hospitals with the same achingly familiar sad symptoms: anxiety, fearfulness, chronic low self-esteem, and depression. Women who bought the myth of fulfillment-through-others find themselves mired in a situation in which these debilitating symptoms thrive. Anxiety is a natural by-product of other-directed people whose sense of self-worth depends on pleasing others. Fear of the outside world makes sense when we realize that women have been systematically deprived of dealing with real world concerns and have been denied access to skills that would enable them to cope with common adult/male situations: travelling alone, buying a car, taking out a loan, or applying for a job. Chronic low self-esteem is a built-in consequence of the traditional female role. Lack of recognition for female skills and qualities, internalization of "negative" female traits, and feelings of inadequacy with respect to adult skills and behaviors leaves no foundation on which to build a sense of self-worth. Depression, the number one mental health problem for women, is understandable and perhaps even appropriate when seen as a response to the real insoluble dilemma many women find themselves in. Feelings of dissatisfaction and disappointment that grow out of unrewarded role demands cannot be explored or expressed, for to do so is to bring into question one's adequacy as a woman. Since a woman cannot entertain the idea that satisfaction and fulfillment may be obtained by meeting her own needs, she must resign herself to live within the confines of the traditional female role, coping with gnawing doubts about her adequacy as a woman. If resignation is a basic and major ingredient of depression, then many women are depressed because they see no way to alter their circumstances.

Alice is an example of a "female identified" woman. When Alice entered therapy, she was ridden with anxiety and guilt and was afraid of speaking in groups and being in crowds. She felt she had failed utterly as a wife and blamed herself for her childrens' problems. She saw herself as an emotional "basket case," plagued with feelings which she felt were wrong and which she could not control. She had little confidence in her adult skills and abilities (despite her good performance as a graduate student and 20 years of managing a large household). Like so many women, she felt "bad" when she was direct and forthright.

Like her mother, whom Alice saw as the perfection of womanhood, she tried to put the needs of others before her own, to avoid conflict, to control her "negative" feelings, and above all, to control her anger. Alice feared her tyrannical father. Her mother seemed willingly submissive to him and was unable to defend her daughters against his arbitrary and capricious bursts of anger and violence.

Alice married a man who was more like her mother than her father. He was a highly-respected professional, very passive, indirect, and unable to express his feelings or even his personal opinions forthrightly. In Alice's words, spoken with a combination of awe and resentment, her husband was a "very nice man."

Within a few years, Alice found herself in a small town with three small children and a workaholic husband. She felt isolated, abandoned, and overwhelmed with responsibility that she felt was hers alone. Feelings of dissatisfaction blossomed into resentment which soon found expression in sarcasm, blaming, and periodic rages that left her reeling in self-recrimination. She began to hate herself as an ungrateful nagging wife and failed mother.

The pattern established between Alice and her husband during this time hardened over the years. Feeling attacked, wanting to avoid conflict at any cost, not knowing and perhaps not wanting to do anything, scared, yet quietly judging, her husband withdrew more and more. Alice felt she had driven him away with her anger. Her anger grew out of her dissatisfaction with her role and with her husband. She could not give validity to these dissatisfactions, much less recognize and take responsibility for them, because this would put her needs and wants on a par with those of her husband and children. To Alice, thinking of oneself as worthy of equal consideration was selfishness and a cardinal sin.

When Alice came into treatment, she had already begun on the long road to resolving the double bind split. She had become aware of deep unresolved feelings; she had begun to explore the sources of her unhappiness; and she had acted on her need to find a vocation by returning to school.

Still, she was deeply humiliated by her feelings, particularly feelings of vulnerability and anger. She saw herself as defective for having these feelings and both hated and admired her husband for his ability to remain emotionally unscathed.

During the course of therapy, Alice began to appreciate and revalue her female skills: her sensitivity, perceptiveness, her ability to be empathic and understanding, her warmth, good humor, and her ability to care for others. The most difficult thing for Alice was to value her feelings, to accept that her ability to feel strongly could be a source of strength, and to understand that each feeling had its source in life and not in her defective female psyche. Alice also had trouble remembering that she had the right to take her needs and wants into account and that doing for oneself did not automatically bring harm to others.

When therapy stopped, Alice had separated from her husband, finished graduate school and began working full-time.

The "Male-Identified" Woman

Despite tremendous pressure to adopt the traditional female role, there are and always have been a small group of women who resisted that pressure and opted for the other alternative, the traditional adult/male role. These women exude well deserved self-confidence as they are usually successful at whatever they try. They are self-directed, have confidence in their ideas and beliefs, are not afraid to speak up, and are willing to take risks. They have faith in their problem-solving abilities, and pride themselves on their independence. These women find their satisfaction and fulfillment in identifying *with* men (excelling in traditionally male skills and emulating traditionally male attitudes, personality traits and behaviors) rather than *through* men. They reap the rewards of this identification by feeling effective in society and valued for what they do.

This powerful though small group of women are often viewed by other women with a mixture of awe, suspicion, and scorn and are seen as "exceptions" by men who learn to deal with them as equals. The most outstanding feature of this group is their disassociation from their female selves. Unlike their "female identified" sisters and those women who feel split between adulthood and womanhood, these women do not feel devalued or unappreciated for their "positive" female qualities. Rather, they seem to see themselves as inherently lacking in these female skills and have no desire to cultivate them. Neither do they struggle to control their "negative" female traits because, like men, they have denied and suppressed them. Since they share society's mistrust of emotions, they do not see how emotions are a valuable source of information about themselves and others. They are not tormented by feelings of vulnerability and helplessness, and are unaware of their strong needs for connectedness and intimacy. They do not worry about their ability to "make it" in the "real" world because that is the arena of their expertise. Because their self-esteem is built on their image of themselves as self-reliant, objective, reasoning, competent persons, they tend to overestimate what they can do and feel crushed when they need to ask for help or reevaluate their plans. Like many men, what causes them to begin to evaluate their chosen role is a crisis or pressure from a mate.

Kay was in crisis when she began therapy. She was in pain, and her feelings were close to the surface. After the demise of a long relationship in which she had been the strong one, Kay decided that the way to feel good again was to start a new life. She left her hometown, sold her house and business, left her network of friends, and took off for a city where she knew no one and had no idea what she would do. Kay had always made it on her own, and she believed she would do it again. After a couple of months she started to "fall apart.'' She became very emotional, crying a lot, and fearing situations that had not bothered her before. Her self-confidence was eroding and with it her image of herself as a problem solver. Kay's grief over the loss of her lover invoked old feelings of vulnerability from childhood abandonments and could not be tolerated. She had learned early to survive these losses by forbidding herself to feel them and by denying her need for support and comfort. Her grief was something to be solved, to be gotten over as quickly as possible. The way she had done this in the past was to "move on" to something new. This time it had not worked.

Kay reluctantly reached back into her childhood to answer my questions. She tried to present her childhood experiences in a matter-of-fact way, but my spontaneous responses of dismay and sadness took her aback. Tears began to form. It was as if, for the first time in her adult life, Kay was seeing her childhood for what it was: characterized by abrupt and unpredictable changes, pockmarked with losses, and peopled with adults who could not be relied on or trusted.

Kay's mother had left the family when she was two. She and her two brothers were left with her father, who struggled to support them. At age six, the family broke up. Kay was sent to board with a neighbor family. From this point on, she was constantly on the move. She estimated that she made between 15 and 20 moves between the ages of 6 and 17. Throughout these years, Kay returned periodically to her father, who was having more and more difficulty coping with life and who had developed a severe drinking problem. Kay described her father as an emotional, loving but inadequate and passive man. She was his favorite. She worked with him in the family auto repair business and developed confidence in her abilities to learn new skills, work hard, and manage things.

In helping Kay learn to value her feelings and needs, I first had to convince her that it made sense to do so. I pointed out that her unmet needs and unclaimed feelings affected every aspect of her life—her choices, the quality of her relationships, and her behavior in general. I told her that I understood how important it was for her to feel in control of herself and how frightening it was for her to feel so overwhelmed with unexplained and unwelcomed emotions and needs. I argued that one cannot control something whose existence is denied. I suggested that she could achieve control of her life by acknowledging her own feelings and needs instead of denying their reality.

Using this approach with a "male identified" woman serves two purposes. First it earns her trust because it reassures her that you can be respected as a clear thinking, logical person. Second, it allows her cognitive self to give the "go ahead" to explore the uncharted territory of her emotions.

Slowly Kay began to understand that it made sense to acknowledge her needs and feelings. She learned that feeling did not render her incapable of thinking and that in acknowledging her vulnerability, she became stronger. During the course of therapy Kay began to cultivate some of her own "positive" female qualities such as empathy and a real perceptiveness about people. She also began to own and respect some of her "negative" female traits such as vulnerability and emotionality. In learning to value the female side of herself, she began to value women in a new way. This process was accelerated by Kay's growing involvement in the women's movement where she began to identify with other women rather than seeing herself as separate and apart from them.

This group of "male identified" women have tremendous potential. When they are able to combine their adult skills and experience with a new found sense of value in their female skills and qualities, they offer a model of wholeness to other women. They hold out the possibility of integrating adulthood and womanhood: a healing of the double bind split.

Women in the Middle: The Split

Another group of women, rather than making a primary identification with either the adult/male or female pole of the double bind split find they must struggle to incorporate both. However, instead of combining the aspirations, needs, and traits from both the adult/male and female role models, they feel they must choose: choose between their desire to be effective, competent adults and their desire and need for intimacy and connectedness. They are trying to get both but are trapped in the double bind which requires women to choose between personal effectiveness and affiliation.

The women in this group have good adult skills developed from experience in living independently and testing themselves in new situations. They value and admire adult/male attitudes and personality traits and often appear to those who know them casually to "have it all together." They are self-sufficient, strong, sensible, and adventurous, but they doubt their own ability to cope and worry that their competency is a facade that could be shattered at any time. They are terrified of their vulnerability, of their profound need and desire for nurturing and support, which they associate with weakness and womanhood. Unlike "male-identified" women, they are not disassociated from this side of themselves but only too keenly sense the urgency of their needs and feelings.

While attempting to control their feelings of vulnerability and to maintain their facade of competency, they are also gauging how far they can go in presenting themselves as capable self-directed people. Though they wish to be respected as effective adults, they are afraid to fully demonstrate their abilities, voice their opinions and ideas, and in general, stand up for themselves. They have difficulty in making their needs known and in setting clear limits. When differences arise, they tend to doubt their own perceptions. Disagreements thrust them into a conflict situation where all the options seem to have negative consequences.

As these women are afraid of exposing their vulnerabilities and emotions—their "negative" female traits—they are equally afraid of exposing their strength and personal power—their adult/male skills and traits.

An area of strength for the women in this group is their well-developed "positive" female qualities. They are sensitive and perceptive and have superior ability to empathize with, and understand the needs, feelings, and experiences of others. For women caught in the split, utilizing these "positive" female qualities is an almost foolproof way to get rewarded and to avoid the uncertainties that accompany more self-defining behaviors. It is hard for them to say "no." They feel guilty when they put their needs first and have great difficulty in asking for their needs to be met. In relationships they set themselves up as givers but become resentful and angry when their needs go unnoticed and unmet. They worry about their seeming incapacity for intimacy. They do not understand why they feel diminished in intimate relationships or why they feel more intact when they are not committed to one person. Yet they are also afraid to be without a relationship for very long.

Women caught in the throes of the double bind conflict are pulled in opposing directions and their behavior reflects this tension. Because they have internalized contradictory messages about who they should be, they swing from one extreme to another, coming to a halt in the middle where they remain immobilized and unable to act.

Marcia came into therapy thinking that she needed a couple of sessions to help her come to a decision about whether to remain in her current relationship. A couple of sessions became four years as Marcia's ongoing struggle to resolve the double bind emerged as the major issue in her life. Marcia had internalized the double bind dilemma and it affected two problem areas in her life, "love and work."

Marcia is the youngest of five girls in a Catholic family in which the traditional male/female roles were vividly played out by her parents. From her mother Marcia developed an image of the "ideal" woman: a "madonna" figure, who was warm, loving, unselfishly giving, modest, understanding, pleasing, and yet desirable. Her mother put the needs of her husband and family first, did not complain, kept her emotions and insecurities to herself, and was never demanding, possessive, jealous, or overtly angry. Marcia adored and idealized her mother, a "good woman" who seemed to possess only the "positive" and none of the "negative" female traits. This ideal was reinforced by her father, who referred to her mother as a "saint" and publicly commented on her virtues and beauty. Her father's explicit opinions and her mother's consistent behavior gave Marcia clear, specific, and powerful messages about who women are and how they should act. She learned that a woman's most powerful asset is her good looks, that women derive their value and power from male approval, and that men approve of women who are beautiful, passive, and giving.

Three factors kept Marcia from making a straight-forward identification with her mother and becoming a "female identified" woman. The first was her own basic nature. A large and central part of Marcia's personality was ambitious, adventurous, questioning of authority, striving for independence, and desperately wanting recognition as a competent person in her own right. These strivings were modeled by her father, the undisputed boss of the family. To Marcia he represented action, knowledge, intelligence, sophistication, excitement, accomplishment, control, and independence. The part of Marcia burning to claim her own personal power, yearned for her father's permission and recognition of her own aspirations and accomplishment. She learned instead that such desires were "off limits" to her as a female.

The second factor was that Marcia saw cracks in the maternal picture of the "good woman." She noticed that her mother was often tense and anxious and suffered from periodic bouts of depression. A disturbing contradiction began forming in her mind: why should a "good woman," my mother, who is so loved and adored be unhappy? As she got older, Marcia decided that her mother's unhappiness was caused by the fact that she was not in control of her life, and she began to resent her mother for allowing her father to control her. She came to fear and abhor the submissiveness she saw in her mother, in other women, and in herself. For protection, Marcia cultivated a facade of independence and competence which successfully hid her female weaknesses and vulnerabilities.

The third factor was that Marcia knew, primarily from her father and her mother's treatment of him, that while the world may adore and cherish women in their place, it really valued men and all that maleness stands for. Marcia could not stop herself from wanting a "piece of the action." The problem was that Marcia could not bring herself to go after what she wanted. She could neither enact her male aspirations nor accept her female expectations. To choose either of these mutually exclusive alternatives was to experience consequences that were unacceptable to her. To opt for enacting her adult/male aspirations carried the threat of ultimate aloneness. This was based on the fear that "if I am myself, no one will want me." Marcia felt that if she acted on her own needs and desires, she would automatically be choosing to give up the opportunity for a long lasting relationship. On the other hand, to opt for choosing to live out her female expectations meant giving up her goals and dreams, putting herself second, and accepting the idea that her happiness must come from the successes of others. Like so many women caught in the opposing currents of the double bind dilemma, Marcia often found herself immobilized in the middle: anxious and ambivalent, unable to act on her own needs and desires, and unable to commit herself to an intimate relationship.

Marcia's relationships with men caused her the greatest anxiety. Armed with the message that affiliation with a man was the only acceptable path to happiness and excitement, Marcia was never long without an ongoing relationship. Once involved, she would begin to resent her partner's accomplishments, knowledge, and what she saw as his male prerogative to come and go and do as he wished. Her female expectations demanded that she always maintain the facade of the "good woman," catering to the needs, desires, and interests of her partner to the exclusion of her own. Her ensuing resentment culminated in an overwhelming feeling of being trapped. When these feelings became too strong, Marcia would precipitate a "separation crisis." These separations allowed Marcia to experience a sense of power and separateness which she could not achieve within a relationship. Slowly, Marcia would allow her partner to re-enter her life and the cycle would begin again.

The other area affected by the double bind conflict was work. Marcia was hampered in finding a vocational direction by old messages and experiences which created a conflict between her personal desire for achievement and her need for affiliation. She felt she could not, on her own initiative, make her life involving and interesting. During a hiatus between relationships, Marcia faced up to the fact that only she could make her life meaningful and exciting. In a haze of self-doubt, she slowly completed her BA, and to her amazement, graduated Cum Laude. After much deliberation, Marcia decided to go to business school. This choice was influenced by her desire to be part of a traditionally male profession where there would be no dispute about the value of her work and by a desire to work with women, using business skills as a tool.

Marcia's struggle to bring together the "male" and "female" parts of herself was still in process when she decided to end therapy. She had come a long way toward unravelling the disturbing contradictions in her behavior and understanding the source of her ongoing anxiety. She developed confidence in her ability to achieve and had taken great strides toward accomplishing her lifelong ambition of becoming a competent person. Though it was still difficult for her to define her limits with people and to express her needs and desires to her new boy friend Bill, she was much more aware of the cyclical process that the suppression of her needs engendered.

HEALING THE SPLIT

The ways women adapt to the double bind are influenced by their individual personalities, life crises, and circumstances. Throughout our growing-up years we have experiences that continue to shape the kind of adaptation we will make to the double bind. As adult women our lives and our choices reflect the adaptations we have made. Alice fulfilled her female expectations by marrying "well" and trying to mold herself into the ideal wife, mother, and homemaker. Kay chose relationships where she was the strong, competent one, and Marcia enacted her "split" adaptation by dropping out of college at 19 and marrying a man who she felt embodied those adult/male traits that were "off limits" to her as a female.

Though our adult adaptations to the double bind are riddled with tensions, frustrations, and a sense of incompleteness, we continue to use them till they fail utterly to be effective in coping with life. Any number of things can precipitate a breakdown of the old mode of adaptation. In Kay's case, it was finding herself alone and frightened in a strange city, facing the fact that her well thought out plans and coping abilities had failed her. We often pick up the thread of our client's lives at such points of disequilibrium, when they are vulnerable, in pain, and are motivated to face the unworkable adaptation.

The beginning phase of therapy is like a see-saw: one week of awareness followed by two of confusion and denial. The therapist's understanding of the double bind and the struggles it poses for women will help her remain patient, accepting and compassionate. This is also a time for the therapist to learn about her client's unique double bind dilemma, how it developed, and how it has operated in her life.

The first three steps in the healing process are part of any long-term therapeutic endeavor. These are: 1) becoming aware of one's defenses and learning how they operate; 2) understanding what the defenses are protecting; and 3) becoming aware of how one's present behavior is connected to past experiences and old unexamined assumptions and beliefs. I will focus on the next 3 steps which pertain specifically to healing the double bind split: 4) revaluing "positive" female qualities; 5) redefining and learning to value "negative" female qualities; and 6) reclaiming and developing adult/male skills and qualities. The seventh and last phase of the process is learning to enact one's new found sense of wholeness within the context of society as it is. These phases of the healing process overlap, and the issues they raise continue to be dealt with throughout therapy.

Revaluing "Positive" Female Qualities

Women who have spent most of their adult lives primarily identified with the traditional female role often feel that they have been doing nothing. The therapist must question this assumption, and in exploring with her client what she has done over the years, it will become obvious that she has accomplished many things and acquired many skills. It is helpful, when possible, to point out a skill that is transferable to the world of paid work.

It is also devastating for "female identified" women, who usually disdain their "negative" female traits and feel deficient in adult/male skills and abilities, to believe that they have failed in the societally sanctioned female role. This is a good place to begin building self-esteem. As the woman begins to trust and value what she already knows, she will begin to build a foundation from which she can take some risks and treat herself more gently and respectfully.

For Alice, learning to value her "positive" female skills and traits was the beginning of the healing process. Once Alice could see that she had done a credible job in raising her children, running a large household and performing the many obligatory duties of a college professor's wife, she realized that she had acquired many skills that could be used in running her own life. This opened the way for her to consider the possibility of leaving the marriage in which she had felt trapped for 25 years.

Redefining and Learning to Value "Negative" Female Qualities

This step involves helping women acknowledge and respect the abilities to be vulnerable, to rely on others at times, to accept and affirm weaknesses as well as strengths, and to be emotional.

Learning to value the so-called "negative" aspects of femaleness is difficult because our culture is so profoundly mistrustful of these feeling states which are seen as destructive, as having the power to take over and control. Women, like Marcia, carefully conceal these negative feelings under a guise of independence and competence, or like Alice, deride themselves for possessing these awful qualities.

For Alice and Marcia, the process of appreciating and respecting their emotions and vulnerabilities was the most difficult part of the healing process. Both women were deeply ashamed of this part of themselves, but each dealt with it differently. Alice accepted these "negative" traits as an inevitable consequence of being female, was able to admit these feelings, and to express them openly. This enabled us to explore the genesis of her feelings and make conscious a general issue or a specific instance which had given rise to her feelings. This was extremely useful because it helped Alice de-mystify and eventually trust and value the information her feelings generated. Alice began to see her husband's lack of emotion, not as a source of his strength, but as his way of protecting himself from his own insecurities and fears. This understanding allowed Alice to

let go of the vicious cycle of anger at her husband for his lack of
emotional responsiveness, guilt for having confused and upset him,
and humiliation for having exposed herself once again as a weak
over-emotional woman.

In contrast to Alice, Marcia dealt with her "negative" female
qualities by trying to deny them, yet her fears, doubts, and insecurities were always present. As hard as Marcia tried to exorcise
these demons, she could not rid herself of them. Helping Marcia
find value and strength by acknowledging and accepting her
"negative" female traits was only partially successful. Her shame
at having these traits and her need to have me see her as competent
and "together" made getting at her needs, fears, and insecurities
very difficult. Marcia felt that if she continued to bring up her fears
and anxieties it meant that she had not made progress. This made
her feel that she was indeed hopelessly weak and that I would
become as disgusted and judgemental of her as she was of herself.
While this revelation opened things up a bit, Marcia continued to
struggle with her dreaded weaknesses. Though Marcia left therapy
still tending to hide behind her well composed facade and still often
rejecting and deriding herself for her weaknesses, she left therapy
more accepting and more self-confident than when she started. This
was due primarily to her integration of the sixth step of the healing
process.

Reclaiming and Developing Adult/Male Skill and Traits

In order for women to feel like whole people, they need to recognize and have confidence in the adult/male skills they possess, to
believe in them, and in some cases, remember and reclaim the skills
they once had but lost.

In working with women like Marcia, it is important to help them
recognize that they are, and have been running their lives by themselves. They are, in fact, the independent competent people they
present themselves to be. They need to close the gap between who
they really are in the present and their old internalized childhood image of who they are. The therapist can: encourage independent
thinking, show interest in, and respect for personal views and opinions, support risk taking, reinforce goal setting and decision making, and point out the discrepancy between current functioning and
outdated self-image.

With women like Alice, it is important to search for examples of risk taking and help them recall and then reclaim old aspirations and discarded goals. It is also important to help them name a few of the real world skills concealed in their devalued female role.

In helping women develop the adult/male traits of assertiveness and directness, the fear of violating the female injunction to please must be addressed. Each assertive action, every attempt to be direct and clear, poses a mini identity crisis, a close encounter with the double bind. Both Alice and Marcia wrestled with this problem. Both Alice and Marcia saw the men in their lives as stronger and more powerful than themselves, yet they felt that the smallest assertion on their part could not be handled by their men and would cause them to crumble, retaliate, reject or abandon them. It is helpful to bring this contradiction to awareness and to ask women to examine its truthfulness. In Marcia's case, such questions helped her separate her boyfriend's actual behavior toward her from her learned expectations of male behavior.

Most important for women to understand is that their fear of enacting their adulthood is grounded in reality. Once women can see that they are faced with an externally imposed dilemma, they can begin to see the possibility of a solution. This solution must involve embracing all of who they are and ignoring the societal imperative to choose between adulthood and womanhood. In this context, trying new adult/male behaviors becomes an experiment in personal growth and a challenge to an oppressive belief system aimed at keeping them stuck in the quicksand of the double bind.

Enacting One's Wholeness Within the Context of Society as It Is

The main work of this period is helping women find new structures to meet new needs based on a new-found commitment to wholeness. This means taking responsibility for making hard choices about living, loving, and working.

For Alice this meant deciding where she wanted to live and what kind of place she wanted to live in. She experienced the excitement and trepidation of moving to a new house in a new neighborhood, knowing that this decision was hers alone.

Kay was faced with the decision of whether to enroll in the PhD program of her choice. This time her choice included an assessment of her feelings and needs, and she did not fool herself into believing that the move would be easy and painless.

Marcia, who through most of therapy was ambivalent about living with her boyfriend, finally decided to buy a house with him, knowing that she would continue to struggle with her need for intimacy and her need to feel separate and whole.

Though clients leave therapy at various points in the healing process, some come to a natural end point. For those who reach this point, this can be an exciting phase of therapy. It is a time to summarize and consolidate, to explore options, take risks, and enjoy feeling good about oneself. It is also a time to face, often with a sense of sadness and disillusionment, some of the larger themes that claiming one's wholeness and taking responsibility for one's life bring to the fore.

The feminist therapist is keenly aware of the importance of maintaining a non-hierarchical relationship between herself and her client. This ending phase of therapy is a time when the client's self-knowledge and awareness cause the relationship to move in the direction of full equality, mutual respect, appreciation and enjoyment. For the therapist, it is a time to enjoy the person her client has become, and to savor the intimacy that grows between two people who have taken a long journey together and have grown to know each other well.

REFERENCES

Broverman, I. K., Broverman, D. M., Clarkson, F. E., Rosenkrantz, F. S., and Vogel, S. R. Sex Role Stereotypes and Clinical Judgements of Mental Health. *Journal of Consulting and Clinical Psychology,* 1970, *34,* 1-7.

Laing, R. D. *Self and Others.* New York: Pantheon Books, 1969.

Miller, J. B. *Toward a New Psychology of Women.* Boston: Beacon Press, 1976.

Women and Anger in Psychotherapy

Alexandra G. Kaplan
Barbara Brooks
Anne L. McComb
Ester R. Shapiro
Andrea Sodano

As a group of feminist therapists working together in a clinical setting, the authors of this paper are firmly committed to a therapeutic modality which would counterbalance the prevailing cultural disapproval of female anger. Women's anger, we are unambivalently convinced, needs to be recognized, validated, and confirmed. Whatever the final form of expression of this anger, we see the acceptance of the *feeling* as one of the primary goals of our work. But as we shared the details of therapy hours with one another, what emerged was quite different than we had intended; apparently we, ourselves, had real difficulties dealing forthrightly with our clients' anger. There were several occasions when the reporting therapist "did not hear" the client's anger that was so apparent to the rest of us. At other times, the therapist's own defensive patterns would

Alexandra G. Kaplan is Associate Professor of Psychology, as well as Research Associate and Co-Administrator of Counseling Service at the Stone Center, Wellesley College. Barbara Brooks is staff psychologist at Hawthorne Cedar Knolls School. She received her degree in clinical psychology from the University of Massachusetts, Amherst. Anne L. McComb is a psychologist in private practice in Amherst, Massachusetts. She also provides consultation and evaluations around issues of child abuse at a community mental health center. Ester Shapiro is a clinical psychologist in private practice, specializing in clinical work, consultation, and writing on family development and development of parenting. Andrea Sodano is a clinical psychologist in private practice. She also supervises and trains Psychology students and interns and co-ordinates an employee assistance program at South Shore Mental Health Center, Quincy, Massachusetts.

This paper is based on a symposium presented by the authors and Susan Pinsker, Leigh Schonitzer and Barbara Fibel entitled "Women and Anger in the Therapeutic Relationship" (Alexandra G. Kaplan, Chair, 1978). The presentations from which the present paper was derived included: Barbara Brooks, Women's powerlessness as it affects anger in the therapeutic relationship, Anne L. McComb, Women and anger in the sex-role differentiation process, Ester R. Shapiro, Anger between women in the therapeutic relationship: A developmental perspective, Andrea Sodano, The effective use of the woman consultant's anger.

become activated precisely at those times that she, herself, was dealing with unrecognized anger of her own toward the client.

Putting our feminist principles into action took more than a personal commitment. This recognition was difficult, but made manageable by the fact that similar problems emerged in the work of each of us. Thus, we realized that the essence of the problem was not in the individual therapist, but in the fact that despite our training, individual therapies and value orientation, we still carried with us remnants of the same cultural proscriptions against anger which we had so readily anticipated in our clients. Working on the topic of women and anger in therapy, then, meant attending to the nuances of anger as they related to historical *and* interactional dynamics. It also meant grounding our inquiry in specific sociocultural conceptions of female anger as these become manifested in therapy for our clients and ourselves. This paper will first address some of the more pertinent sociocultural forces and then illustrate their translation into our clinical work.

THE CULTURAL SHAPING OF FEMALE ANGER

The prevailing proscription against female anger can best be understood within the broader context of women's subordinate role in society (Miller, 1976). As subordinates, women's economic and emotional survival is dependent on the support of the dominants. Thus, it becomes crucial that women develop in ways that do not threaten this support. In general, this means that women learn to be sensitive to the emotions of others, and to pay special attention to those qualities that maintain and enhance relational ties. These qualities become a central part of women's self-concept, evolving into what can be called women's *relational self* (Gilligan, 1982; Miller, 1982; Jordan, Kaplan, & Surrey, 1982). Women's development occurs within a relational matrix, and women's increasingly complex and sophisticated relational qualities form one important aspect of their sense of identity and self-esteem.

This developmental paradigm contains some major positive components. By including in their *self*-development the capacity to foster and enhance relational development, women play a primary role in facilitating the growth of others—a quality essential for the survival of society (Miller, 1976). Ideally, women's pursuit of their own needs and their freedom to develop a full range of affect and expression would be fully consistent with the primacy of a relational self. That is, there is nothing *inherently* threatening to one's connectedness to others in one's own self-development. But all too often there is also a price that is paid for this relational development. Women's capacity for "agency"—the ability to act so as to further their own needs and wishes—is responded to by others as threatening to relational ties. This response easily becomes internalized, so that women, themselves, may experience agentic qualities as threatening to their relational self. Further, in its worst manifestations, women may even lose the capacity to identify what their own wishes are, apart from how these are defined by others.

One of the primary losses within this pattern is women's capacity for assertive behavior in general, and the direct expression of anger in particular. The expression of anger can come to be equated with precipitating loss, not just of another person, but more importantly of a key component of one's self-esteem—one's capacity to maintain relational ties. To the extent that this equation exists for individual women, it can lead not just to the distorted or deflected expression of anger, but to a lack of awareness of the feeling of the anger itself.

Mothers and Daughters

The translation from cultural paradigm to individual psyche is mediated through the family, beginning with early parent-child relationships. Under current social arrangements, in early infancy this typically means the relationship with the mother. In general, women's relational self produces an intense and intimate bond between mother and infant. But within that context, mothers attach to and become especially identified with their infant daughters (Chodorow, 1979). This identification enhances the mother's wish to recreate herself in her daughter, but also to mother the daughter as she, the mother, would like to have been mothered. There is great variation from one mother to the other as to the power of these two pulls. Cutting across most mother-daughter relationships, however, is an enhanced responsiveness to one another, a growing sense of mutuality and shared concern. At first, this is primarily from mother to infant daughter, but increasingly the daughter, as well, internalizes her mother's "capacity for concern" (Winicott, 1965).

Thus, the infant daughter's early training in expression of anger occurs within the context of this bondedness. Perhaps the first critical stage in which this training becomes salient is the rapprochement subphase as described by Mahler (1968). It is at this time that the daughter consciously tries out her differentiation from the mother. This contains the joy of power and competence, but also the possibility of abandonment and resultant helplessness. All too typically, it is the daughter's manifestation of power and competence in forbidden territory that brings on mother's anger and stimulates the fear of abandonment. This fear, we must remember, is especially powerful for the daughter, for whom the state of connectedness with the mother is an integral part of her growing sense of self. Thus, we have a situation in which mothers must set realistic limits to their daughters' movements out into the world. To the daughter, however, mother's displeasure creates two reactions. First, it communicates to her that she has disappointed mother, a position inconsistent with her growing wish to please and gratify her mother. Second, it stimulates in the daughter a fear that mother's anger will signal a lessening of the all-important bond between mother and daughter. The impact of these two reactions on the daughter, not surprisingly, is to modulate her misbehavior so as to please the mother. To the extent that rage has been included in the mother's definition of "misbehavior," this, too, will come to be curtailed.

The "Angerogenic" Milieu

If it were only the mother's reactions that contributed to the daughter's inhibition of anger, this inhibition would not be nearly as widespread a situation as it seems to be. What happens, however, is that themes which have their origin in the early mother-daughter relationship are repeated and supported by the daughter's growing relational network as she moves psychologically first into the larger parameters of her family, and then into the immediate world beyond.

Within the immediate family, there is a strong likelihood that the daughter will be the recipient of, and/or witness to some form of verbal rage or physical violence from parents. Frequently cited estimates suggest that violence of some sort within the home is found in close to 50% of American households regardless of socioeconomic status or ethnic background. Fathers contribute disproportionately to this violence, being responsible for over half of the instances of child abuse and virtually all of the spousal abuse. Thus, in many cases, the daughter's fear of her father may augment or dominate her reactions to her mother's disapproval. The inhibition of one's own self-striving is much the same, only now it is out of fear of debilitating consequences, rather than fear of abandonment. Daughters can receive a clear message, then, that self-expression, including the expression of anger, may be attempted only at great risk to the self.

If women were being raised in a culture in which there were few or isolated instances that were anger arousing, and in which the absence of anger were the general norm, then the inhibition of women's anger would not be problematic. However, neither of these situations is the case. It is this conflict between female development and current cultural exigencies which creates distress. In fact, women's position in contemporary society is one in which there are systematic, predictable, consistent situations which are potentially anger arousing. Much has been written and spoken in the last few years about the economic and interpersonal oppression of women, and need not be repeated here. What needs to be stressed, however, is that each specific instance of an oppressive pattern— lack of opportunity for job advancement, fear of physical abuse, insults to one's intelligence—all tap into and can potentially fuel the fires of anger. Women live in an "angerogenic" milieu. The process of suppression of rage is a constant one, as is the fear that the anger may somehow "leak out" at the expense of women's sense of self in relation to others.

In addition, women live in a society in which anger is as American as the corporate executive and a pitcher of beer. That is, anger is a fundamental, accepted and frequent experience of a large segment of the American population—men. This anger may be expressed verbally, or acted on in forms of violence, frequently against women. Our culture has no systematic, reliable process for containing male violence. Thus, at the same time that women feel disconfirmed and invalidated by their anger, they observe that for men anger is self-confirming, self-enhancing and supported by the social order. Paradoxically, this observation becomes yet another source of anger which must then be discounted, disowned and denied.

Women, then, live in conditions in which the experience and expression of anger can be a threat to their sense of self and their sense of security with others, at the same time that they are surrounded by conditions which can potentially evoke this disconfirming rage. At base, it is this tension between the anger-evoking conditions of women's lives and the forces which encourage and suppression of anger in women that forms the core of work with anger in psychotherapy.

WOMEN, ANGER, AND PSYCHOTHERAPY

Until recently, there was only a small body of literature on the general topic of working with anger in psychotherapy, and even less on anger in therapy with women. Fortunately, this situation is being redressed. Psychotherapy has been recognized as a legitimate forum for women to explore the place of anger in their lives (Rice & Rice, 1973). In particular, Miller (1983) has carefully delineated the process by which anger in women becomes inhibited, and the emotional difficulties that result. As noted above, any psychotherapeutic work with women and anger must take into account the cultural and interpersonal forces which stimulate anger in women and the forces which serve to suppress it.

Women vary in the extent to which they can bear what Andrea Dworkin (1976) calls the "agony of being fully conscious of the brutal misogyny which permeates culture, society and all personal relations." The therapist can help her client decide to what extent and in which situations she wishes to remain in touch with this anger, and when in touch with it, how, if at all, she is comfortable expressing it. In a society where women are so pervasively oppressed, each woman must be aware of the limits to her energy. If she is to be effective, she must learn to be selective in her individual expression of anger at that oppression.

Psychotherapy can also provide a forum for a woman to explore her fears and other feelings about the expression of such anger, and the availability of other human resources to support her attempts. Finally, in this endeavor, as in others, therapists and clients can learn to accept responsibility for their actions. Through trial and error, however painful, women may gain a social awareness which will serve them (and us) well in the battle against the demoralization of women by their roles.

Helping a woman sort out her angry feelings in both her individual and sex-role differentiations also allows her a greater understanding, and thus potential control of her anger. Many clients have come to therapy sessions believing themselves crazy because of the intensity of their anger with a spouse, an employer or even a news item. Helping a client determine how much of her anger is due to an isolated instance of maltreatment, how much to her sense of having often been placed in similar situations by her parents and how much to the fact that this particular incident is a culmination of weeks or months or years of having her adult needs ignored by society, allows the client an important, reassuring perspective on the intensity of her anger. It is also an important ingredient in the client's decision as to whether, and how to express her anger. In this way, she can learn when an expression of anger constitutes a waste of her time and emotional energy, and when such an expression will be psychologically liberating and perhaps even socially or politically effective.

Specific issues can arise around female clients' anger at their mothers. In talking about this anger, women clients often portray a feeling of having been bitterly betrayed by the person they grew up caring about the most. The therapist may need to point out that some of this bitterness is misplaced and belongs instead to the culture in which the mother was socialized. Conversely, the therapist may also need to suggest that the client is attempting to minimize her very real, appropriate anger with her mother by consistently empathizing with her mother's oppressed condition. It can be problematic for a woman to feel a bonding with her mother if it occurs at the expense of her own individual growth. In this way, we encourage the client to experience her genuine anger at her mother while at the same time recognizing the cultural factors underlying her own and her mother's lives, actions and emotions.

The process of differentiating while still maintaining the relationship between mothers and daughters has strong implications for the relationship between the woman client and woman therapist. As part of the simultaneous pulls for closeness and differentiation, the client may wish for the therapist to be the perfectly responsive mother of her infantile wishes, who handles smoothly this fine line between nurturing and letting go. This request can only be frustrated by the therapist, because of the constant tension between these two dimensions. Depending on her own history, the therapist may sometimes err on the side of offering overwhelming or intrusive nurturance, or may err on the side of distancing, giving the client autonomous space which the client is too vulnerable to use and which she experiences as rejection.

If as therapists, we become the self-sacrificing mother, we will likely expect our clients to improve in return—an expectation which would serve to undermine our therapeutic work. We may then begin to feel depleted, uncared for and unappreciated by this ungrateful child. Mother the martyr, is a familiar character in many of our family histories; we know from experience that we expect compensation, whether the price we ask be guilt, nurturance in return, conformity to an approved image, or self-aggrandizement. And we will be angry if we do not receive compensation.

Alternatively, the therapist may attempt to be the distant, competent mother; we may feel frustrated by the client's insistent needs for closer, nurturing support and dismayed by her dependent clinging or demands for care. This is particularly likely for us as professional women who have made it through school at the expense of the free expression of our own needy feelings. The more uncared for we feel in our own lives, the more difficult it will be for us to respond sensitively to our clients' needs for care.

A client who has learned to give up power and control in exchange for intimacy may do so in therapy, and then become angry at her resulting feelings of helplessness and dependence. She may feel that the therapist, like her mother, wants her infantilized in order to care for her. This will at some point lead to an angry battle for control of the therapy, as the client attempts to win her right to grow as an autonomous person. Again, too much nurturance may feel like loss of control, but too much distance may feel like rejection and abandonment. The battle often ensues when the therapeutic work moves to a particularly painful and difficult issue for both the client and the therapist. The therapist's attempts to support exploration may feel to the client like being pushed out of the nest.

In a difficult and painful, not to mention angering, therapy relationship, one of us began work with a client who joined her in an intense family identification. Lisa had requested a female therapist because her relationship with a male therapist hadn't worked out, "You know how stubborn men can be." Lisa came from a tremendously enmeshed family much like the therapist's own, including a deep symbiotic attachment to her two sisters and mother, and an overtly angry relationship with her competent, professional father. She found it much easier to be angry at her father than at the women in her family, yet her therapist felt that Lisa's unacknowledged anger at women was the central issue in her work toward independent functioning and more adaptive expressions of feelings. The therapist felt that Lisa needed support for autonomous action, and began by giving her a great deal of space for exploration, particular-

ly of her anger at her husband. Lisa found anger intolerable, preferred to turn it inward rather than express it directly, and was
sometimes dramatically self-destructive. At the same time, the
therapist was attempting to protect herself from enmeshment with,
or engulfment by this especially needy client. Lisa experienced this
as rejecting, and asked her not to be the distant therapist in a variety
of ways, including escalating suicide threats and imagery.

The therapist eventually responded to Lisa's requests for help, including her request for drugs, by initiating an emergency session
and setting up a consultation with a psychiatrist, as well as halting
the attempts to help her explore her anger. Lisa was initially
grateful, but also began to feel infantilized and soon became critical
of the help she was being offered. She saw the therapist as having
abandoned her to a man, as her mother and sisters had done, and
dealt with these feelings by now seeing the therapist as a well-
meaning but incompetent friend. Her willingness to nurture Lisa
had transformed the therapist into Lisa's critical and incompetent
mother from whom she had to protect herself. Lisa turned the anger
toward men, which she had begun to acknowledge and explore, into
an escalation of her attempts to leave the therapy. The therapist was
soon furious with her, but felt unwilling to express her feelings
directly, or even to acknowledge their full weight. She recognized
that she, herself, had in part been responsible for her client's anger
by having overresponded to the client's stated wishes for assistance,
without at the same time recognizing the client's ambivalence about
receiving such help. Thus, the client responded to the threat of the
therapist's intrusiveness by increasing the distance between them,
ultimately leaving the therapy.

Therapists may also demonstrate the same ambivalence between
closeness and differentiation expressed by the client just described.
As female therapists, we may be vulnerable to a wish to maintain
our relationships with our female clients and thus be unprepared to
recognize our client's healthy growth, which can and should lead to
termination. At the same time, there may be a tendency to resent the
client's presentations of helplessness, which place excessive demands upon the therapist. Both of these conditions—moving away
and moving toward—if felt as intrusive or excessive may stimulate
anger in the therapist, which has more to do with her own personal
issues than with the ongoing, actual client/therapist relationship.

Hopefully, the therapist will recognize the inappropriate nature of
her countertransferential response. Such a recognition may leave

the therapist feeling unprofessional and vulnerable, a stance which is likely only to increase her self-protective reactions vis à vis the client. A preferable position would be for the clinician to balance her appropriate professional "objectivity" with what Miller (1976) has called two of women's greatest strengths: the ability to be vulnerable and thus to grow, and the ability to care about and do for others and thus to help them grow.

The interplay of cultural, interpersonal and intrapsychic dynamics can be illustrated by the work which one of us did with a young adult woman. Betty entered therapy with a long history of depression. A college graduate, she had few friends and worked nights in a small business. In the initial phase of the work, Betty was distant and exhibited neither tears, anger nor sadness appropriately. She expressed great concern over her inability to "know" what was real in her interaction with other people. She had, she said, a tendency to misperceive and distort reality. For example, she had been molested by her father during her adolescence, but she sometimes doubted the validity of this memory.

Working with Betty, it appeared that beneath her flat affect there was a great deal of potential rage. As a way of defending against her anger, she would question her perceptions in ways that led to significant distortions. The exploration of the anger behind her distorted perceptions, its subsequent recognition and its effective expression became major issues in her therapy.

In the early sessions, Betty denied any anger though she was often hurt by others. She didn't get angry with her roommate who tracked snow through the living room, who refused to do her share of the household tasks and who in general made Betty's life uncomfortable. Instead, Betty blamed it all on herself: perhaps she should be more understanding. Like many of us, she had developed the sense that her life should be guided by the constant need to attune herself to the wishes, desires and needs of others. She never confronted her roommate for fear of hurting her feelings or making her angry. This way, Betty felt "safe"—after all, her roommate didn't know she was hurt. At this point the therapy focused on the inhibition of anger, its dynamic underpinnings and its present manifestations.

Several sessions later, Betty cancelled a session just ten minutes before it was due to begin. On this particular day it was the only appointment the therapist had. But Betty had to do something for her mother, so how could the therapist be angry? They spent the next session exploring Betty's unconscious motivation, her anger toward the therapist and her inability to state her needs when they conflicted with the wishes of someone else. A supervisory hour helped the therapist to recognize her own anger, with its countertransferential elements, and her reluctance to state her own needs, if only to herself, so that she could have better taken them into account in working with Betty. But she still assumed that her unrecognized anger had had no impact on their previous hour.

Imagine her surprise and chagrin when, at the next session, Betty reported feeling "strange" with the therapist. Encouraged to talk about their last contact, she recalled that at that time she had felt that the therapist had been distant: according to Betty, this was just another example of her own tendency to misperceive reality. The therapist, recognizing the clinical importance of confirming Betty's perceptions, acknowledged that she had indeed been angry with Betty at the time, and that her own unawareness of the feeling had created the "distance" that Betty had correctly perceived. Following this critical interchange, Betty began to make significant strides in trusting in her own perceptions and delving more deeply into the process of self-exploration.

CONCLUSION

Women's developmental paradigm, in which preservation of the relational self plays a central role, can serve to inhibit agentic action and the expression of anger. Thus, it becomes especially pertinent for psychotherapy to counterbalance this direction. But this same developmental paradigm can prevent therapists from recognizing and exploring anger in a female/female therapy dyad. The intensely interpersonal nature of psychotherapy both stimulates feelings of anger that may have been a part of earlier, intense relationships, and inhibits its exploration to the extent that this triggers fear of loss. For clients, this may result in relational swings between closeness and distance, as each is ultimately frustrated by the therapeutic process, which in turn generates anger and a reversion to the opposite pole. For the therapist, countertransferential defenses are likely to interfere with the recognition of her own and her client's anger, and/or her effective handling of her own feelings toward the client. These patterns can be alleviated through a careful understanding of the cultural origins of these dynamics, and specific attention to the ways they may interfere with the ongoing therapeutic work.

REFERENCES

Chodorow, N. *The reproduction of motherhood.* Berkeley: The University of California Press, 1979.

Dworkin, A. *Man hating.* New York: Dutton, 1976.

Gilligan, C. *In a different voice.* Cambridge: Harvard University Press, 1982.

Jordan, J., Surrey, J., and Kaplan, A. Empathy and the female self: Implications for therapy. *Work in Progress: A series of working papers,* 1982, 82-02, The Stone Center, Wellesley College, Wellesley, Ma.

Mahler, M. *Human symbiosis and the vicissitudes of individuation.* New York: International Universities Press, 1968.

Miller, J. B. *Toward a new psychology of women.* Boston: Beacon Press, 1976.

Miller, J. B. The construction of anger in women and men. *Work in Progress: A series of working papers,* 1983, 83-01, The Stone Center, Wellesley College, Wellesley, Ma.

Rice, J. K., and Rice, D. G. Implications of the women's liberation movement for psychotherapy. *American Journal of Psychiatry,* 1973, *130,* 191-196.

Winnicott, D. W. *The maturational process and the facilitating environment.* London: Hogarth Press, 1965.

A Legacy of Weakness:
Unresolved Issues
in the Mother-Daughter Arrangement
in a Patriarchal Culture

Joan Hamerman Robbins

*A mother's victimization does not merely humiliate her, it muti-
lates the daughter who watches her for clues as to what it means to
be a woman . . .The mother's self-hatred and low expectations are
the binding-rags for the psyche of the daughter.*

A. Rich, 1976, 243

*And the one doesn't stir without the other. But we do not move
together. When the one of us comes into the world, the other goes
underground. When the one carries life, the other dies. And what I
wanted from you, Mother, was this: that in giving me life, you still
remain alive.*

L. Irigaray, 1981, 67

THE LIMITATIONS OF OUR CULTURAL CONDITIONING

For as long as we can remember, and our mothers and grandmothers can remember, we have lived in a patriarchal world. Our
interior world is profoundly influenced by our history; thinking,

The author, co-editor of this book, is a feminist therapist in private practice in San Francisco, and on the editorial board of *Women & Therapy*.

I wish to acknowledge the influence on my own thinking of the writings in this issue of P.
Caplan, J. Heriot, A. Kaplan, and J. B. Miller. My work would not have been possible
without theirs.

language, consciousness itself have all been informed by a patriarchal value system. Our social experiences growing up female reinforce low self-esteem, passivity, limited expectations for ourself;
and encourage dependence on males for our self-worth and sense of
accomplishment.

Intertwined with this is our female biology: the menstrual cycle
and our reproductive capacity. We live close to a body rhythm that
reminds us of the possibility of being taken by surprise and losing
control, themes often translated in our male-defined culture as
weakness, fragility, inadequacy.

To acknowledge these issues is to recognize the depth of our oppression—psychologically and culturally. We resist seeing the
power of culture to define and limit us as females; it is safer to hate
mother than to see how *we* are also shaped and molded by forces in
the culture that have shaped and molded her experiences. Both
mother *and* daughter exist in a shared subservience to the rule of the
father.

Unresolved issues in the mother-daughter arrangement came into
sharper focus when I began to notice that a group of my female
clients were all blaming their mother for not providing them with a
different set of experiences while growing up. These women did not
see the part that culture and father have played in creating and
perpetuating a value system that denies female experience.

My clients grew up in the traditional Caucasian, middle-class
family of thirty-five years ago. Father was hard working and successful; he provided adequately for the family. Father was the link
to the world outside the home, a world which suggested excitement
and adventure to a small child. As described, the mothers were
depressed and unhappy, tired, lacking zest for their lives. Most of
them had three children within the first five years of their marriage
and have functioned in their adult life as wife/mother/homemaker.

A Legacy of Weakness

In this paper I have selected aspects of my work with five women,
quoting from them as they illustrate the patterns of the legacy of
weakness. As I observed distinct patterns began to form. The principal pattern reveals a woman who describes herself as inadequate
and stupid. This woman cannot see what she does do because she is
always focused on what she does not do. Unresolved childhood
themes of helplessness get expressed in the adult woman's belief

that she is stupid, helpless, incompetent. These feelings are not hidden, they are openly expressed. What is masked is an unconscious high standard for performance and success which is at odds with the expressed low self-esteem. The demands this woman places on herself are impossible to meet—another confirmation of how inadequate she is!

A second pattern details a strong, competent, independent woman who is stubborn, critical, perfectionistic; always demanding more of herself. This effective stance conceals an internalized concept of failure and inadequacy. These apparently very different women are struggling to avoid what I call a "legacy of weakness."

The legacy is handed down through the female side of the family: grandmother, mother, sister; it is ancient and complex. At its most primitive, the legacy is a yearning for closeness and affection, for the caring, nurturance and dependency associated with early childhood. Because this yearning is ancient it feels enormous. In girlhood each woman learned to deny and repress these strong feelings because to experience their intensity meant you were inadequate, weak, female! It is imperative to keep this vulnerability repressed.

Mother, the principal donor of the legacy, is viewed as a needy woman. She is described as: "cold," "a shell," "empty," without her own identity. The need to reject mother is clear, the feelings she generates in the daughter are so threatening.

> Karen: "Mom taught me not to do what was hard. I remember when I was learning how to roller skate I had trouble learning to stop, and Mom said, 'Give it up!' "

> Miriam: "The barren landscape of my Mother—it's so stagnant, infertile, nothing grows there. It's all gray and brown—actually those are colors I like—but it's not a nurturing environment. How I wish it were different. I want my Mother to be a model for me. How can I be okay if she isn't?"

Father

Father's role is very important in how the legacy is passed down from mother to daughter. In a patriarchal culture father holds the promise of more. This girl becomes aware of father's power and confidence and she is attracted to these qualities. Interlaced with these themes are memories of erotic feelings between the child and father that can play a part in how the girl is drawn to her father's influence. In therapy strong feelings emerge. Father is the favored parent, more real and alive.

> "When he came home things began to happen, it was fun. I don't ever remember having fun with Mom."

> Anna: "Dad was the center of attention in my family; all three of us 'girls,' Mom, my sister and I, vied for his attention—you could never get enough of it. I remember how my Mother would call us in from playing to change our clothes before he came home for dinner, so we would look pretty for him. And how we loved that! Dad was everything positive, he heaped a lot of love on us—he was a real King."

> Julie: "My Father was all over the place, blustering, bullying, butting in, we could never do anything without his knowing all about it. He dominated all of us, there was no sharing, he controlled everything. Mother had no control over anything, it was always what Daddy wanted."

The Psychological Limitations of the Alliances

In exchange for father's affection and attention daughter shifts her allegiance from mother to father. Mother begins to be viewed as a helpless and inadequate person in the child's efforts to become a "big girl" and ally with father. Mother and female values are rejected; father replaces mother as the child's role model. This shift deeply affects the child's emotional connection to being a girl. Important sacrifices are made in this shift: no matter how hard daughter tries to model herself after father neither of them can really ignore that important difference—she is female.

Additional significant sacrifices are made in this alliance with father which are *both* at the expense of the child's relationship with her mother and her expression of infantile needs. Daughter begins to devalue maternal closeness and in this move away from mother begins to repress her infantile needs for nurturance and dependency which we can presume had been met by mother. Deep and important issues about intimacy, the expression of feelings, and femaleness are effected in the turn to father. In the intriguing economy of the psyche, with profound reinforcement from culture, the girl learns to equate overwhelming feelings with being female—both of which are devalued in our culture.

The pulls are out of balance; decades of oppression have taken their toll. Mother cannot compete with what father has to offer. In addition to being totally nurturing, she is expected to be adequate, competent, responsible, creative, assertive, etc. Obviously this is impossible! The child is seeing the exhaustion of the mother without awareness of the protected role culture has assigned father in the family. He does not stay home; he does not participate in the daily care of the child, nor does she see his struggle in the world.

The daughter's turning away from mother produces a reciprocal withdrawal by mother. The child experiences this as mother's coldness and emptiness. Yet the daughter is ambivalent; she pushes mother away, but wishes that mother would tug back. If mother would tug back, daughter would know she cared!

> Thirty years later Miriam says: "I want to tell her way down deep inside it hurts. It feels like you didn't care. I'm angry with my Mother for what she never gave me. I don't feel as if there was substance there, someone to bounce off of—anything would have been better than the nothing I felt."

> Julie: "Mom tolerated everything, she never got angry or said a harsh word; she was never physical with me. She didn't hug or kiss me, or play with me like Dad did. She is quietly there, but I need her to be more active. I need her to engage in controversy with me—I need that for my own sense of who I am."

It is speculative, but possible that mother is pushing her girl to be more assertive, independent, less clinging. This is mother's way of helping her daughter to grow up and become more of a person. Given the influence of patriarchy mother can presume that the female way to wholeness is through the father; a daughter who has her father's blessings may have an easier life.

The presumption that a heterosexual choice will be made early in childhood is another deep value in our culture; this is as powerful a cultural imperative as is the assumption that males are more valued than females in our society. It is possible that the homophobic fears, a cultural legacy we all share, gain added reinforcement by the manner in which mothers train daughters to heterosexuality. These pressures complicate the already devalued bond between mother and daughter.

The Complex Unfolding

There is much confusion. A perfectionistic stance is cultivated as a way of handling the pressure to adapt in order to survive and grow. Belief in one's own ability and capacity to weather inner and outer events is diminished. Low self-esteem and limited expectations affect our sense of adequacy and keep us dependent on males.

> Karen, a research biochemist, is working on these themes. She learned from her Dad, the favored parent, that love is earned by being perfect. She was rewarded and acknowledged for doing well in school; disciplined or humiliated when she did not excel. In therapy Karen realized that she becomes numb when she is confronted with making a mistake. Karen said: "At work if an experiment fails I feel I have to quit. I can't allow any room for error. It is hard to tell anyone about this. Mistakes were not allowed in my family. I feel like I am wading into feelings of despair and helplessness. I want to get right out! If I were a perfect person I'd have this all figured out by now. If I'm not perfect I'm not lovable. In my family, you belonged by being perfect."

In our culture females are trained to believe that men know more than women. We can certainly appreciate why Karen is drawn to men who are perfectionistic and in control. Her boss and her lover always seem to know what Karen should do and do not hesitate to tell her this. Their assertions protect Karen from her panic about making a mistake.

The absence of an adequate role model in our mother coupled with a domineering father does profoundly affect our ability to be responsible for ourself. In therapy talking about her boss, Miriam realizes: "I don't want to get angry and speak up for myself, it reminds me of how much I wanted my Father to do it for me. Dad did everything, he always acted like he knew what to do; and he could do it better, certainly better than Mom—and I believed him. Mom plays a part here too, she was always critical of me, called me a spoiled brat, felt I always got my way so she didn't offer me advice or choices, just criticism."

> I sympathize: "You will have to find your own way and it can be damn hard."

Miriam: "Yes," (teary) "I feel a deep wish for someone else to be there with me, helping me do it. Yet I know it's all up to me—and I hate knowing that. Dad taught me to be tough and sharp and never let on if you feel weak—feeling weak is a terrible admission. Mom was always weak, she never stood up to my Father or fought for herself. If only once I could have seen her stand up for herself. I hate her spinelessness!"

New Experiences in Therapy

Therapy with these women is a delicate and complex working through of old, painful, long repressed feelings from childhood that have been denied and devalued because they are reminders about one's femaleness. The working through centers around the new female-to-female bond that can become a reworking of the mother-daughter arrangement. Because that bond has been vehemently attacked we can anticipate that the client-therapist arrangement will be constantly tested. Keep in mind the mistrust of female closeness, it comes up over and over in the therapy and is at the heart of what is being repaired.

Susan grew up in an affluent family; father is a very successful, domineering person; mother is described as a "shell." During Susan's childhood her parents took many trips away from home. She and Michelle, her older sister, were left with the nurse. Susan expressed her feelings: "It was fun without them—and I knew they'd come back."

When Susan was four something different happened. The girls were sent to summer camp while the parents went to Europe. Susan remembers disliking it at first and crying a lot; finally she was placed in Michelle's bunk. She is still angry at Michelle who at six, could not be a BIG sister and make it okay for Susan. After a time, Susan remembers it got to feel better; thirty years later, she is determined to stay with her mastery of this event. "I really did make it, and all other separations from home have been easy."

There is a lot of pride; I have appreciated that, impressed with her ability at four to handle a difficult situation. I have also been trying to educate Susan to the possibility of other feelings, like hurt, anger, betrayal at being left in a strange place for a long time. Susan has listened to me as if I am speaking a foreign language, ready to fight with me. She said, "I sense you want something from me and I'm not going to give it to you." Of course I want something, I would like her to make contact with those old feelings. If Susan were to feel this event she would know she missed her mother, that she was frightened and alone and did not like it!

This year after we each had a vacation, Susan announced she wanted to interrupt therapy. During her vacation Susan realized she works hard and decided to reduce the pressures in her life. She and I had already had the experience of two separate journeys in therapy, we know the work can be picked up at another time.

> It was important for Susan to experience her own pace, and my support of her decision. With the freedom to choose for herself, Susan became very perceptive about what remained for another time. She said: "I am aware that I am holding on to a magic nugget about separation. I don't want to feel those feelings now. I want to save something that's singularly mine for myself—I'm not ready to integrate that yet."

Many issues have become clear in writing this paper. I realize that I, too, admire women who are strong, competent, and successful. Getting caught in this adaptive stance has made it harder for me to recognize the fragility that is being masked. I have frequently overestimated the strength of my client to deal with her inner feelings.

> Miriam walks into therapy looking very sad: "Other people have a life, I have nothing. I can't get committed to anything. It feels like I'll never change or make a career for myself. I'm living out my Mother's life, and my Father's life; nothing ever mattered—all that negativity. No one gave me a reason for doing."
>
> Miriam is angry, sad, stuck. We get another glimpse into a pattern we have noticed before—her waiting for someone else to give her a push. I asked her if she was mad at me for not pushing her more. Hesitantly, Miriam becomes angry. "I do want you to be more confrontive, tell me what to do; this is my first experience with therapy, I don't know if I'm doing the right thing. I want more direction from you. I have this image of one big session in which I get angry and tear the room apart,

and then it's all fixed. It is so slow. I am angry that I only see you one hour a week. You don't know what the rest of my week is like.''

I accept Miriam's feelings, validate her anger that there isn't more for her. Notice again the dilemma: Miriam is waiting for someone else to do it for her, not yet able to take responsibility for herself—which adds to her belief that nothing is happening in therapy. The following week we get more clarity. Miriam continues to be angry with me. ''I felt you had expectations for me; you wanted me to be this goal-oriented career woman. Can't you see how stuck I am in being a two-year-old!'' When Miriam finished I reflected my feelings back to her: I felt trapped. I recognized her wish that I have expectations for her because it would mean there is hope. Yet I knew that if I had ambitions for her she would be furious with me.

Miriam responds: ''It's my own fear that I am stuck in my life and I'll never change.''

I continue: ''There is confusion in finding our way. We do stumble and grope; it is not always clear. Yet, I wonder, are we avoiding your fears of getting close and committed to the work?''

Miriam sighs: ''Maybe I don't need to protect myself so much.''

Further Refinements in the Work

The work affords me a continuous opportunity to rethink issues. Occasionally, a piece of important work is close to new understanding when the client expresses the wish to come to therapy less often. Sometimes the request coincides with my vacation or her vacation, the summer, money problems, an increase in pressures at work, or school, or home. Often this same woman will take a long vacation from therapy to return years later and continue her work.

I respect the client's right to determine the course of her therapy. Nevertheless, at times I experienced anxiety and confusion when my client expressed her wish to alter the regular pattern of appointments. I felt concern when my ''clinical'' judgement did not match her ''personal'' judgement. Upon reflection I believe the client was trying to teach me how to respond to her needs in a manner that does not ignore mine, and also validates her perceptions of self. I am learning how to match and respect her rhythm, so she can experience the "optimal distance" at which she feels safe practicing separation and individuation within the view of a caring person. We are reworking "rapprochement" in a new arrangement between women.

At times I feel I am walking a tight rope. This woman is exquisitely sensitive to exposing her old pain and hurt. But we are doing it: slowly, carefully, wading in and out of despair and hopelessness, growing stronger and more self-assured as we proceed. Perhaps the most profound modeling is going on in the ancient wellspring where we discover repressed feelings. By staying close, being available and unafraid of feelings I demonstrate that a woman can be soft and vulnerable *and* competent and skilled—a new fusion of female talents.

On our journey toward wholeness we must step aside from our conditioning. In order to be accepted by the culture we have learned to reject vulnerable feelings which we have associated with our mothers. Perhaps now we can stop blaming mother and begin to take responsibility for ourself. We are all subject to periods in our life when we feel dependent, vulnerable, scared; we can also anticipate times when we feel strong, competent, adequate, alive! To be human means to be subject to an incredible range of feelings.

REFERENCES

L. Irigaray, "And the one doesn't stir without the other," *Signs: Journal of Women in Culture and Society,* Vol. 7, No. 1, Autumn 1981.

A. Rich, *Of Women Born: Motherhood as Experience and Institution,* New York: W. W. Norton, 1976.

Between Women: Lowering the Barriers

Paula J. Caplan

INTRODUCTION

Virginia Woolf called the realm of relationships between women "that vast chamber where nobody has been" (Rich, 1979). These relationships have only recently become the subject of psychological inquiry. In 1977, I began to investigate the societally imposed obstacles women have to overcome in order to form supportive friendships or reasonable working relationships with each other (Caplan, 1980, 1981).

The more we investigate the barriers between women (Arcana, 1979; Dworkin, 1974; Rich, 1976; Dinnerstein, 1977), the more we find we have not so much ourselves and other women to blame but rather the entire sexist structure of our society (Firestone, 1970). We are further discovering how extensively, how pervasively the traditional, sexist forces in society have emotionally blackmailed our mothers, and us as mothers, into repressing our daughters; for it is in that earliest, most intense of relationships—the mother-daughter one—that so many of the barriers between women have their roots. In this paper I will briefly outline some of the sources of these barriers as they lead to difficulties in two of the primary problem areas for women today: in the workplace and in the interaction between

The author is Associate Professor, Department of Applied Psychology, Ontario Institute for Studies in Education; Assistant Professor of Psychiatry, Lecturer in Women's Studies, University of Toronto; Coordinator, Canadian Psychological Association Section on Women and Psychology.

An earlier version of this paper was published in Paula J. Caplan, *Between Women: Lowering the Barriers* (Toronto: Personal Library Publishers, 1981). Reprinted by permission of the author.

51

feminist and antifeminist women. (More barriers, including the fear of sexuality between women, are discussed and explored in more detail in Caplan, 1981.)

We begin with the fact that females are supposed to be patiently, endlessly nurturant. Society instructs families to raise their daughters to conform to this stereotype, and "families" has usually meant "mothers," since they have done most of the childrearing. This has often meant that mothers were so busy training their daughters to *give* nurturance that the daughters did not *receive* as much as their brothers. This process was aggravated by the fact that strict limits on what women were allowed to do, and what feelings they were allowed to show, left the mothers feeling angry or depressed. Often, women feeling lonely and frustrated turned to even their very young daughters for support and understanding, or for taking over the parenting and housekeeping tasks they felt unable to do. Little girls put in the "little mother" position have then grown up with many of their own needs for nurturance unmet, thereby set to fall into the same pattern with their own daughters. Such girls grow up resenting women who do not meet their emotional needs. The nurturant female stereotype has a related consequence: because we do not expect men to be nurturant, we are often unduly grateful for the slightest shred of warmth and support offered by males but, in sharp and unfair contrast, we feel that even a nurturant woman (or mother) could give us more "if she wanted to." Thus, we undervalue what women do.

In a more general way, society requires mothers to teach their daughters to place more value on the friendship, opinions, and judgment of men than on those of women. Even before their daughters are born, more mothers still hope their first child will be a boy than a girl.

Another barrier is formed by the set of rules and constraints to which little girls are more subject than little boys: "Don't run around. Don't get dirty. Cross your legs. Don't get angry. Don't be sexually active. Don't be so aggressive." These prohibitions usually come from the mother at the same time as she is telling her son, "I love to see you run around, climb that tree, and stand up for your rights when that other kid tries to bully you. You're a *real boy!*" The little girl watches her mother treat her and her brother differently. But it's not even that simple. The little girl, frustrated and constrained, is being rewarded by her mother when she follows those rules; for the sake of winning her mother's approval, she learns to accept the constraints. Her mother, meanwhile, for the sake of winning society's approval, continues to impose the constraints; after all, the mother is a female and, as such, was raised to work for approval, too.

Females' similarity, both physically and in the way they are classified according to gender, sets many barriers between them. One example is the adolescent's fear, as she tries to suppress her increasing sexual and aggressive feelings, that her mother sees her struggles, knows her thoughts. This originates in the child's belief that grown-ups can read her mind, but it has some basis in fact: our mothers know what it is like growing up female. Mothers, therefore, probably know or sense the presence of the still-forbidden sexual and aggressive feelings in their daughters. Since a primary task of adolescence is separation and individuation from the parent, this understanding—which can be a blessing—is often experienced as a curse, an intrusion. This tends to set women on guard against each other.

There are two basic ways to lower these barriers. One requires major social change: Stereotypes need to be abolished, fathers need to share in childrearing, sons need to be taught to nurture, and daughters to be more self-respecting and assertive. In the meantime, change can take place on a day-to-day level, one individual to another. We can be vigilant, watching for signs of these deeply-rooted barriers and of our inclination simply to disparage other females rather than to recognize these tendencies as signs of the misogyny that pervades our society.

As we think about lowering these barriers at this time in history, two areas are particularly important ones on which to focus. One is the interaction of women with each other in the workplace, and the other is the interaction of feminist with antifeminist women. Throughout history, each wave of feminism tends to elicit an antifeminist backlash. The one that became prominent in the late 1970s and early 1980s takes a well-organized and financially an extremely well-funded form. This makes it a particularly strong force that can keep women on opposite sides of that "vast chamber where nobody has been." A similar pattern can characterize the relationships between female clinician and female client and between women in general in the workplace, if we are not careful. What all these situations share are: (1) the way that women's socially-encouraged need for men's approval can come between mothers and daughters and between women of all kinds, and (2) the way that women's learned undervaluing of themselves and other women can come between them.

WOMEN IN THE WORKPLACE

Females have been placed in a dilemma through most of their development because of two sets of labels provided by society: the seductive-submissive-admiring-compliant kind and the powerful-bitchy-castrating kind. It is hard to imagine that anyone would want to be classified either way. However, society has classified a narrow band of behavior as acceptable for females, and everything else as one of the two types of behavior embodied by these myths. Struggle as they may to overcome this name-calling which takes place in their own heads as well as "out there," women bring these labels with them into the workforce.

It is tempting for women to behave in accordance with the Type One myth, the submissive-compliant one. First of all, it is considered acceptable for females. Second, it is likely to please the men with whom one works. This is important, as we have noted, because most of us feel that the men's opinions are the ones we value. In nearly all offices, factories, and institutions, the men are more likely than the women to hold administrative and other positions of power. Therefore, behaving in the submissive-compliant way is likely to please the men, who are likely to have the power to reward, promote, and grant raises and privileges. Females' upbringing makes this a particularly easy pattern to fall into:

> Many little girls never develop feelings of competence outside the sexual arena. When thrown into a situation which demands more adjustment than they can manage at a given time, they fall back on the only skill they think they have in order to achieve the only security they were taught to seek: the sexual attention of daddy. In a business, academic, or political organization, where arbitrary hierarchies exist, those who have status or power are clearly labeled daddies: boss, president, dean, professor, congressman, mayor, and so on. Naturally the "little girls" head for them (Williams, 1976, p. 50).

Of course, their involvement with the "daddies" at work need not be overtly sexual, although sometimes it is. But even when it only takes the form of flirtation, coyness or instant acquiescence to the daddy's wishes on the woman's part, it makes clear that her primary allegiance is to him.

Pleasing the men in power has often been a sure-fire way to alienate other women, who usually have not had the power. If Margo is submissive and compliant with the male bosses, her female co-workers will not be pleased to notice that she puts all her energy into that endeavor while ignoring them. If Margo treats her female co-workers badly, in order to focus her attention on the men in power, she may be promoted or otherwise rewarded. If Suzanne focuses her attention on concern and cooperation with her female co-workers, they will like her, but she may make no progress within her job. Some choice!

Women social workers, psychologists, and psychiatrists have often found this problem particularly difficult, because their daily work involves such intense emotional stress and strain. Especially after long days of trying to help patients who have many kinds of emotional, financial, and social problems, women find it difficult to balance these frustrations and their sense of powerlessness with the comparative power of some administrative responsibilities usually held by men. Administrative problems are by no means pleasant; but they do not carry with them the sense of helplessness often engendered in mental health workers by difficult patient populations. The frustrations that go with having power simply feel different than those that do not. Women may try to cope with their powerlessness by playing up to the men, who do have the power.

In much the same way that being married to a powerful man provides some compensation for a woman's powerlessness, so does being in favor with the men in charge at work. This drives a wedge between women and their co-workers. (Naturally, some of their co-workers are probably female and some are male, and some problems arise between low-status female and low-status male co-workers; but our focus is on the problems between the women.) Women have often been accused of being jealous of each other, and this is what I am describing here. However, jealousy does not arise simply because two women have to work together, but because the only way most of the women will ever be able to acquire any power (or even a whiff of it) is by currying favor with the powerful men.

I will take another example from the mental health setting. When decisions and recommendations must be made which will have important consequences for patients' lives, there is an additional and serious consequence of these problems: the women professionals accord their own judgments and the judgments of the women with whom they work less respect than the judgments of the male clinicians. The same thing happens in the business world, in factories, and in various institutions. A woman makes a suggestion, and everyone looks to the men in the group and to the leader—who is usually male—for some assessment of the worth of that suggestion. Here is one scenario of this process.

A woman psychologist, Dr. Smyth, was presenting to the other professionals with whom she worked some information about a patient. The patient was a woman we shall call Anne, who was receiving public assistance but had a strong sense of her own dignity. There had been an unfortunate chain of events that might have happened to anyone, but because Anne was poor, a government agency had been able to take her young daughter away from her. The daughter, Miriam, had a chronic illness, and the mother spent all her waking hours caring for her. Anne had few friends and was socially isolated. About every three months, Anne would become overwhelmed by the strains of the physical and emotional care Miriam required; at these times, she left the child with a close relative and spent a boisterous weekend. At the end of the weekend, she would return and spend another three months taking care of Miriam. She had never abused or neglected her Miriam or behaved inappropriately in her presence.

When the government agency, through a series of unfortunate events, apprehended Miriam, Anne was shocked and frightened. Feeling unfamiliar and at the mercy of the court system, she appeared in court and interpreted what happened there as "The agency workers said I'm a lousy mother, and the judge must have agreed, or he would have sent Miriam back to me by now instead of postponing it." The agency's position was that Anne would have to prove she was willing and able to care for the child before they would return her. Due to the complexities of court procedure and evidence, the case was adjourned several times before a decision was finally made. The mother interpreted each adjournment as yet another attack on her mothering ability. Her already poor self-esteem was severely shaken, and with each adjournment she began to wonder aloud whether she was such a bad mother that Miriam would be better off living with someone else.

Dr. Smyth, Anne's psychologist, worked in an office in which a male psychiatrist had to review all of her work. He informed her that the focus of her therapy with Anne should be on getting her to

express what he called "the negative side of her obvious ambivalence about her chronically ill child." He said that her comments like, "Maybe Miriam would be better off without me, since
everyone says I'm a terrible mother," demonstrated her wish to be
rid of the child. Dr. Smyth felt that Anne's feelings were understandable in view of the stress of caring for Miriam and of what she
considered her humiliation in court. She assumed that many mothers
have such feelings, but that does not mean they should be encouraged to focus on that part of their relationship with their child. Dr.
Smyth suggested to the supervising psychiatrist that it would be at
least as important to work on rebuilding Anne's self-esteem. The
supervisor replied that she was allowing her "motherly" feelings to
get in the way of seeing what this patient really needed.

Dr. Smyth's opinion about the appropriate emphasis for her
therapy with Anne was devalued by being classified as a typically
female opinion. Her judgment that the proper course was to work on
the patient's strengths was translated—or mistranslated—into her
supposed wish to overprotect or take care of her patient. This was
interpreted as a sign of her overinvolvement with Anne, an attitude
considered unprofessional.

A woman colleague, hearing both Dr. Smyth's opinion and that
of the supervisor in a group meeting, readily agreed with the supervisor's opinion. Although this woman regularly agreed with the
opinions of the men in the office, Dr. Smyth found it hard not to feel
foolish and inadequate as a psychologist. Later, talking privately
with her female colleague, Dr. Smyth was astonished to hear the
woman not only reverse her position but also do so in a way that
showed she was not even aware of what she was doing. This other
woman responded to the male supervisor's need to be agreed with,
and to the rewards she would get by seeming to side with him.

Women find themselves divided against each other in every kind
of work. If they are housewives, each is so concerned about being a
supermom that she has reason to fear the observing eye of another
potential supermom. In the factory, the office, and the institution,
women may compete fiercely with each other for what little power
may be available to them. When men do that, it is considered a sign
of genuine masculinity, achievement motivation, and striving to
reach the top. When women do that, it's a different story. First,
competing for something other than a husband is considered
unfeminine. Second, the men who compete ruthlessly with other
men have a much greater chance of being promoted, receiving
raises, and acquiring power than do the women who compete

ruthlessly with other women. Let's face it, women have not had much power or much chance of getting it; so, after all their fruitless struggles, they have often found themselves without power, promotions, or raises, and also without the friendship and allegiance of their women co-workers.

Language has been a useful tool in turning both men and women against women who were trying to succeed in the workplace. One might call it a *trick* of language were it not so powerful and pervasive that it has become more of a system for classifying the behavior of men and women, so that—in most cases—the men's behavior could be admired and the women's reviled. Consider the eloquent point this poster makes about how the same behavior is given different names, depending on whether a man or a woman displayed it:

> A business man is aggressive;
> > a business woman is pushy.
> A business man is good on details;
> > she's picky.
> He loses his temper because he's so involved with his job;
> > she's bitchy.
> He follows through;
> > she doesn't know when to quit.
> He stands firm;
> > she's hard.
> His judgments are
> > her prejudices.
> He is a man of the world;
> > she's been around.
> He drinks because of the excess job pressure;
> > she's a lush.
> He isn't afraid to say what he thinks;
> > she's mouthy.
> He exercises authority diligently;
> > she's power-mad.
> He's close-mouthed;
> > she's secretive.
> He climbed the ladder of success;
> > she's slept her way to the top.
> He's a stern taskmaster;
> > she's hard to work for (cited in Eichler, 1980).

A great deal has been written about the Queen Bee syndrome: the woman who acquires a powerful position in a traditionally male-run workplace and does not feel any allegiance with other women or any wish to help them. Heady with the belief that she is a special woman, she feels she has nothing to gain and her special status to lose if she tries to help other women into similar positions. The Queen Bee has not only achieved success in her job but has also done this with the help of males; usually, they put her where she is today so that she has won the approval of the highly valued sex. The Queen Bee is usually described as a woman executive or an under-secretary of some government department, but she exists in every kind of workplace. She may be the first woman supervisor on an assembly line, where she is now expected to drive her former colleagues so hard that they resent her intensely. This was eloquently illustrated in the film, *Norma Rae,* which is about a woman union organizer in a southern United States textile mill.

Any woman who is put in a higher position than other women in a workplace is in danger of becoming a Queen Bee. Usually, it's a man or a group of men who promote a woman, so that she feels grateful and in debt to them. In addition, promotions are intoxicating. From the time we are children, most of us enjoy the feeling that we are better or more special than the others in our group. And so, the boss' secretary is separated and alienated from the women in the typing pool, over whom she now feels superior.

Intimately related to the Queen Bee syndrome is the fact that within many fields, women still account for a small proportion of the workforce. When most workers in a particular field are male, then a given man can become known for the work he has done. For example, in a university department of philosophy, a man may be known as "the philosopher at the University of Smithville who specializes in Aristotle." A male truck driver for a moving company may become known as "the driver who can make the fastest run from Toronto to Los Angeles for So-long Movers." But the rare woman philosophy professor is more likely to become known as "the woman philosopher at the University of Smithville" (or, worse still, "the blonde"), and the woman truck driver as "So-Long's woman." When a second woman philosopher or truck driver is hired at the same place, the first woman's uniqueness is destroyed; so is the label to which she has become accustomed. Then, both women have to try to make their reputations on the basis of their specific work. That is what the men have been doing all along, but it

is more difficult because there are still so few women in many fields
that the eye of the boss is more critically on them than on most of the
males. They have to prove that management or administration was
right to hire them. To women trained to win approval and acceptance by being feminine, the label of "*the* woman here in our
office" is accustomed and easy, compared to the need to prove
herself by her work. Even most women who take their work
seriously and want to prove the worth of their work *per se* often resent the loss of the quick-and-easy label. The other side of the coin is
that being the only woman in a job places a greater burden on her to
prove herself. Both attitudes often co-exist, in varying proportions,
and the woman feels torn between them: no matter what she does,
she feels somehow dissatisfied.

WOMEN AGAINST RIGHTS FOR WOMEN

Much in the news these days is the group of women who have
poured enormous quantities of time, money, and emotion into trying
to defeat the Equal Rights Amendment in the United States and other
legislation which would give women equal rights in other countries.

> The female subculture has actually divided into two camps, the
> feminist and anti-feminist. It is the worst nightmare of the
> feminist movement come true. . . .It is as if, at the height of
> the civil rights movement, a large percentage of blacks had
> suddenly organized to say: "Wait a minute. We don't want
> equal rights. We like things just the way they are" (English,
> 1981, p. 16).

Until recently, so many women have been financially dependent
on men that they cooperated with men in maintaining the fiction that
this was a safe, privileged, sheltered position for women. Millions
of newly single and newly poor mothers are finding out how untrue
this is. Members of both sexes until recently hid from the fact that
women's position might be sheltered but it is not secure. Nothing in
the Equal Rights Amendment would order these women to get out
into the factories and tell their men to stay home; nevertheless, to
hear them talk, you would think that that was just what we could all
expect. I have wondered for some time why some women would so
strenuously oppose the freedom of other women.

As a psychologist, the intensity and rage of these women (whom

I'll call "oppositional") in their struggle to keep other women down suggests to me that some powerful, perhaps even unconscious force is at work.

First of all, let us look at the two reasons these women give for opposing the liberation of other women and the potential liberation of themselves. Firstly, to advocate rights for women is supposedly unfeminine, and secondly, women will lose their privileged positions in society. Let us look at each of these reasons.

What does "It's unfeminine" suggest? It certainly suggests that oppositional women are afraid that if *they* worked for women's rights they would displease their men. But they are also implying that feminists are unfeminine. They seem to be angry at feminists and sometimes go to great lengths to twist what feminists say. Consider what happened when people in the women's movement suggested that women should be free to work outside the home if they chose. Some traditional women twisted that into the fantasy that feminists condemned the homemaker role. They made so much of this that *Ms* magazine took care to run a cover story about the importance of motherhood. This suggests that it is hard for these oppositional women to believe that women can be free to make choices about their lives and still choose to remain traditionally nurturant, as though they cannot bear to think that a woman might do both. Then, too, they accuse the feminists of being anti-nurturant. Some of their anger may be because they regard feminists as unwomanly for not simply saying: "You traditional women know the *only* correct way to live." They interpret this as a denial of the reassurance and nurturance that women are supposed to give each other.

I think oppositional women are terrified of something for which feminists are struggling: that is the freedom to choose, to decide what directions they want their lives to have. The freedom to choose seems so frightening that they must condemn the women who advocate it and call them traitors to their sex. The freedom to choose is indeed scary but for reasons I'll return to in a moment.

What about the second antifeminist argument: "We don't want to lose our privileged position"? There are some realistic fears included in that concern: the fear of being sent off as a soldier to kill and maim the enemy is one. A second is the fear of having to give up the masks and manipulations women have learned to use while on their pedestals, so that they will be seen directly and unprotected. A third is having to face the fact that certain types of jobs are now available to them for which they feel unprepared or inadequate.

But here again we see what is perhaps the fear of choice itself. If she no longer has privilege and the pedestal, then what? The fear of choice is in part the fear of the unknown, which haunts us all. Few of us actually *like* the people who bring us face to face with our fears. No wonder they fight against feminists.

Now, why is the freedom to choose so frightening? We see the effects of this fear all the time. It may be seen most dramatically in the identity crisis of late adolescence and early adulthood. Psychologist Robert White (1967) has asked the question, "Why is it a struggle, a problem, rather than simply an exciting time?" He points out that resolving the crisis, deciding on one's identity, would not cause much anguish or anxiety if we believed there would be unlimited time in which to try other alternatives. But by late adolescence, we know enough about the reality of death that we know we cannot be a firefighter, and a dancer, and a parent, and a bus driver, and a jungle explorer. We know that, in deciding to become a lawyer, we in some sense kill off or give up forever the doctor or the bus driver parts of ourselves. So as we face the freedom to choose, consciously or unconsciously, we confront our own mortality.

Many antifeminist women are "older homemakers whose children are grown and gone, whose lack of job training gives them few employment options, but who expect their husbands' salaries—at whatever income—to protect them from being put out at the mercy of the job market" (English, 1981, p. 16). Giving the example of the rightwing antiabortionist, antichoice movement, English writes,

> The anti-feminist woman is right about one fundamental thing: the other woman's right to have an abortion does affect her. It does something very simple and, to many women, very upsetting: it takes away their ability *not* to choose. Where abortion is available, the birth of every baby becomes a willed choice, a purposeful act. And that new factor destroys the set of basic assumptions on which many traditional marriages have been based. . . .[The anti-feminist woman]. . .is defensive: reactionary in the sense of reacting to change with the desire to return to the supposedly simple solutions of the past. Like going to war or being born again, it signifies an end to complexity. . .(English, 1980, pp. 26 & 28).

Let us consider what many traditional, antifeminist women do in order to avoid acknowledging their mortality and the passage of time. At least four things come quickly to mind:

1. They spend millions of dollars on cosmetics and cosmetic surgery;
2. They spend millions of dollars on tranquilizers and alcohol, to avoid feeling the effects of the passage of time;
3. They become mothers who tie their children to them desperately, so that they can continue to think of themselves primarily as mothers rather than having to wonder how they are changing or what choices they now must make;
4. They cling to lifelong, heterosexual monogamy as an ideal.

All of these are ways to try to deny that time is passing, to try to live as though life were static and as though change did not bring with it the necessity to make choices.

Many anti-feminists have lived traditional lives. In trying to understand their fears, it is useful to think of Erik Erikson's theory of life stages (Erikson, 1959). He described a series of life stages and said that, although each stage is characterized by some particular issue, all of the issues are present in some form at each stage. Without going into the details of the early stages, what is relevant here is that he describes the next-to-last stage of life as the one in which people are concerned with what he calls the tension between *generativity* and *stagnation.* Generativity includes both reproduction and childrearing, and the productive or creative use of one's other abilities. Erikson says that in the last stage the focus is on the tension between *integrity* and *despair.* Erikson argues that one's sense of integrity in the last stage depends greatly on the extent to which one has in the previous stage found expression of a range of one's abilities and talents. That is, as we face the end of our lives, we feel proud and satisfied with the way we have lived if we believe we have used our generative and creative powers.

Now many traditional women have not felt that they could express any aspects of themselves except those that were, or appeared to be, focused on the needs of others. Many never made choices about the directions their lives would take, except in the form of choosing which man to marry. The other choices were made for them, first by a society that said, "You must marry and have children (and we will judge your value accordingly)," and later by a husband who made the major decisions, and decided whether or not she would be allowed to work outside the home. Many husbands who have agreed that their wives could do something other than childrearing have streamed them toward activities that were, in fact, still nurturant and supportive, such as women's auxiliary groups (which were auxiliary to the primary professional or social groups of the husbands). Or, they were pressured to join groups that still kept them in the nurturant role, such as church groups or volunteer organizations that worked with the disadvantaged. This is not to say that women have not enjoyed some of these activities or to deny the tremendous good they have accomplished. I wish simply to point out the limitations and the lack of choice that were often involved.

An area of study in psychology that focuses on what are called "outlaw relations" has made some interesting observations. An "outlaw relationship" is one that I have with a person who comes from another kind of life and whose values and ideas about what is important are very different from my own. One researcher studied two groups of people: some who had had an outlaw relationship and some who had not. MacPherson (1980) found that people in the former group had a stronger sense of their own identity, of who they were and what they needed, than the latter group. She also found that those who had had an outlaw relationship seemed to have a better tolerance of ambiguity than those who had not. The more secure we are about who we are, the less we are shaken by encountering someone who is different from ourselves, and the less we panic when confronted with new possibilities and choices that we had never before considered. Antifeminists seem in this sense to be "outlaws" who are to be avoided.

Although Erikson has asserted that a woman's identity comes from knowing who will "fill her inner space"—whose wife and whose mother she will be—his theory leads us elsewhere when we think about women's actual experiences. A person who has not been generative or creative in any part of her life outside of raising children and responding to the needs of others, might well find it hard to face her approaching death with integrity. For such a woman, any reminder that she might have made choices about her own life rather than resting in the traditional channel may trigger the despair that is forming in her. The feminist movement and the ERA are certainly such reminders.

There is another source of women's difficulty in dealing with the freedom to choose. They have often been made to feel that they have no choice about their lives and that, in any case, their husbands are far better equipped to make choices and decisions. Jean Baker Miller has pointed out how even extremely capable women believe their husbands have some magical ability and strength that women lack. She says, "This provides their major sense of support. Many women develop a great need to believe they have a strong man to whom they can turn for security and hope in the world'' (Miller, 1976, p. 34). If we never have to make our own choices and decisions, we never have to grow, and we find it hard to know what we want, how we would choose if it were up to us. Germaine Greer (1970) has described the enormous complex of fantasies that are activated by the young girl's first kiss, fantasies that a man will give her life meaning, bring her happiness, and banish her cares. You know the myth: it's Sleeping Beauty, Cinderella, and Snow White. Some of the women who fear the ERA and feminism seem to feel unconsciously that leaving the choices up to their husbands will make it possible to avoid noticing the passage of time and the coming of death; somewhere, deep down, they nurture the hope that their husbands will somehow protect or save them from the unpleasantness the future holds in store, and even, irrationally, from death.

Adrienne Rich's poem, ''Prospective Immigrants Please Note,'' describes the risk involved in choosing something new:

> *Either you will*
> *go through this door*
> *or you will not go through.*
>
> *If you go through*
> *there is always the risk*
> *of remembering your name.*
>
> *Things look at you doubly*
> *and you must look back*
> *and let them happen.*
>
> *If you do not go through*
> *it is possible*
> *to live worthily*
>
> *to maintain your attitudes*
> *to hold your position*
> *to die bravely*
>
> *but much will blind you,*
> *much will evade you,*
> *at what cost who knows?*
>
> *The door itself*
> *makes no promises.*
> *It is only a door.* (Rich, 1967, p. 59)

The intensity and desperation of the antifeminist struggle of these women, combined with its resistance to rational argument, suggest that unconscious processes are at work. The nature of unconscious processes is extremely difficult to prove. However, the evidence is sufficient and what is at stake is serious enough that we need to be aware that these frightened sisters will not listen simply to sweet reason.

REFERENCES

Arcana, Judith. *Our Mothers' Daughters.* Berkeley: Shameless Hussy Press, 1979.

Caplan, Paula J. "Barriers Between Women," *Status of Women News,* June 1980.

Caplan, Paula J. *Between Women: Lowering the Barriers.* Toronto: Personal Library Publishers, 1981.

Dinnerstein, Dorothy. *The Mermaid and the Minotaur.* New York: Harper Colophon, 1977.

Dworkin, Andrea. *Woman Hating.* New York: E. P. Dutton, 1974.

Eichler, Margrit. *The Double Standard: A Feminist Critique of Feminist Social Science.* London: Croom Helm, 1980.

English, Deirdre. "*The War Against Choice: Inside the Anti-abortion Movement.*" Mother Jones, February/March 1981, pp. 16-32.

Erikson, Erik H. "*Identity and the Life Cycle.*" Monograph, Psychological Issues, Vol. 1, No. 1 (1959).

Firestone, Shulamith. *The Dialectic of Sex.* New York: Bantam, 1970.

Greer, Germaine. *The Female Eunuch.* London: Paladin, 1970.

MacPherson, Gael M. "*An Experimental Analysis of the Relationship Between Ego Identity and Outlaw Relations.*" Unpublished B.A. Honors thesis, University of Waterloo, 1980.

Miller, Jean Baker. *Toward a New Psychology of Women.* Boston: Beacon Press, 1976.

Rich, Adrienne. *Snapshots of a Daughter-in-law: Poems 1954-1962.* New York: W. W. Norton and Co., 1967.

Rich, Adrienne. *Of Woman Born.* New York: W. W. Norton and Company, 1976.

Rich, Adrienne. *On Lies, Secrets, and Silence: Selected Prose 1966-1978.* New York: W. W. Norton and Company, 1979.

White, Robert. Lecture at Harvard University, 1967.

Williams, Elizabeth Friar. *Notes of a Feminist Therapist.* New York: Dell Publishing, 1976, p. 50.

Breaking In:
Experiences in Male-Dominated Professions

Beth Milwid

INTRODUCTION

The number of American women in professional jobs has skyrocketed during the past decade. As legal barriers to sex discrimination have been enacted, many women have gravitated toward previously all-male fields.

The media document the achievements of "rising star" and "fast track" women who have advanced quickly, and with apparent ease. "Mary Cunningham" has become a household word. Today, everywhere we turn we see photographs of attractive female executives happily swinging their briefcases, competently chairing high-level meetings in corporate board rooms, or eagerly jumping out of their BMWs to catch last-minute flights. Such publicity would have us believe that for the majority of new professional women, opportunities abound and the path to success is now a blissful one.

Unfortunately this perspective overlooks the psychological realities of day-to-day work life. The truth is somewhat different. Often the beginning professional woman finds that she is the only female in her office. Suddenly she realizes that she has entered into a male work culture and must adapt to it somehow, or fail. Sometimes the woman enjoys visibility and gratifying rewards. At other times she feels harried, discouraged, and out of place. The range of emotions that these women experience on the job is vast. The stresses on the individual can be intense.

During the past decade psychologists and sociologists have started to take a closer look at the daily lives of American working women. Some authors have examined the experiences of individuals who broke into male-dominated professions before the 1970s (Rossi,

---

Beth Milwid is a clinical psychologist in private practice in San Francisco. Her research was conducted under the auspices of the Wright Institute, Berkeley, California.

1965; Epstein, 1970; Hennig & Jardim, 1976). Other researchers have looked at the personality characteristics of female college students who now choose to pursue non-traditional careers (Tangri, 1974; Standley & Soules, 1974; Trigg & Perlman, 1976). A third group of writers has analyzed male-female interactions as they occur in the work place (Laws, 1975; Harragan, 1977; Kanter, 1977; Epstein, 1981).

By the beginning of the 1980s a substantial body of new research had emerged. One set of studies revealed that when women first join the labor force, they confront unique and unexpected psychological challenges. For those who approach male-dominated professions these challenges may involve particular stress and internal conflict.

Before becoming a psychologist, I worked for five years in organizations where I was the only female professional on the staff. At that time I recognized that the pressures I encountered were not unique to me. Many times I longed to share my perceptions with other women similarly employed. I realized then that young professional women need more opportunities to communicate their work experience to one another and to those who can help with strong and sometimes conflictual feelings that accompany beginning career life. I decided at that time that my own research would explore in detail the psychology of women's experiences inside male-dominated organizations.

The following essay summarizes the results of my research. It begins with a description of the study itself and of the women who participated. Next the central findings are presented and discussed. The final section of this paper provides specific suggestions for clinicians who work with female professionals. The unique needs of this rapidly growing population merit the special attention and creative response of all mental health professionals.

BACKGROUND

During the past year I conducted in-depth interviews with 10 bankers, 10 lawyers, and 10 architects in the San Francisco Bay Area. I chose these three groups in order to look at fields that women have entered at rapid, moderate, and slow rates of change respectively. Since I was concentrating on the transition from school into the work world, I selected individuals who had practiced their professions for less than five years.

The majority of women who participated in this study were young, single, and childless. All 30 subjects were middle-class white women in their 20s or 30s. Ten were married, 3 were divorced, and 17 were single. Within the group of single women, six were living with partners. It was striking to note that at the time of this research, only three of the 30 women were mothers.

In connection with these statistics a number of important issues surfaced in the interview material. First, a substantial majority of women reported that they had consciously chosen to defer starting their families until they had completed several years of successful work life. In addition, many observed that their choice of a male-dominated field had meant that this "starting up" period turned out to be far more demanding than they had ever expected. For some women the decision to put off having children was extended again and again into the future.

In a similar fashion, being a feminist and working within predominantly male organizations raised immediate and unexpected challenges for many. Though the number of lesbians in the sample was quite small, nearly half the women interviewed were highly identified with feminist concerns. Individuals in both groups believed that the issues of sexual preference and political activism had grown increasingly conflictual. As they sought to gain credibility and respect with male colleagues, most of the women felt compelled to mask certain aspects of their identities. During the first few years many chose to minimize overt signs of their feminist beliefs.

As a group these women were highly educated, articulate, and sensitive to the complexity of their experiences. Though some were initially ambivalent about participating in the study, most grew intensely involved as the interviews progressed. Several women noted that they were really quite surprised to find out just how much they had to say. Some observed that though they had thought about the special issues confronting women in male-dominated professions, they had never before expressed their ideas aloud.

CENTRAL FINDINGS

The study revealed that bankers, architects, and lawyers all faced a similar set of psychological issues during their first five years. In addition, these young professionals underwent a discrete process of emotional development. Regardless of one's specific job, task, or work environment, the women seemed to encounter the same interpersonal dynamics in almost the same sequence. The following research findings highlight the most salient features of this group's evolution over time.

1. *Work provided a high level of personal and professional satisfaction.*

The interviews showed that in general women in this study enjoyed their work, felt confident about their abilities, and believed that their competence would be rewarded in the future as it had been in the past.

The women were performing well in their new professional endeavors. Their self-esteem was generally quite high.

Most importantly this study produced no evidence that a "fear of success" had inhibited the behavior of women working in male-dominated fields. Quite the contrary, most subjects were very high-achieving professionals.

A district attorney conveyed her sense of satisfaction in the following words.

> I had no idea how fulfilling work could be in the legal world. There really is quite an opportunity to reach one's own personal self-expression. As I looked out at jobs from law school, I felt that they were all in a grid and that I would have to be accepted in some certain way, that I would have to turn into somebody that I was not. I think what's been fulfilling is to find out that there is no such person that you have to become. The great thrill in learning to be a trial lawyer is that there is no one trial lawyer. If a particular job or particular task is appealing to you, then you can do it in your own fashion. I really love this work; it's been really good for me.

2. *Entering a male-dominated profession involved a process of change and development.*

The women were quick to point out that despite this general level of satisfaction, their work experiences had not been without stress. Some cited overwork and physical exhaustion. Others believed that their efforts to gain acceptance from male colleagues had caused them tremendous anxiety, both in the office and at home. Many felt that balancing professional and personal commitments had turned out to be the most difficult and pressing emotional challenge.

Within the sample there was widespread agreement that years one and two had been the most psychologically strenuous. After surviving that initial period, most women found that their work had become more enjoyable and their professional relationships more smooth.

It was striking to observe how bankers, architects, and lawyers all described the same sequence of events that women go through when first beginning life on the job. A maritime attorney offered this advice to young women just starting out.

> Take it on faith that the first five years are very, very difficult and the first one is particularly hard. There really is a lot to experience and the only way you can be experienced is by keeping at it for a while. As far as the difficulty of those first few years goes, it's hard to decide what percentage has to do with being a woman and how much of it has to do with just being inexperienced. The two of them progress together. The experience gets better.

3. *Few women expected any difficulties working within non-traditional fields.*

As noted above, the women went through a clearly defined process of adaptation in adjusting to their new roles. The first step involved their entering into organizations with very few preconceptions about what it would be like to work only with men. It was striking how such a sophisticated group of women had given so little thought to the issues prior to entering the work world. A banking vice president described her lack of clear expectations.

> I always figured I'd end up in a female profession; I never thought about going into business. It was all a total surprise to me. I didn't think I'd work in a male-dominated profession. Actually, I didn't think I'd work much at all. I thought maybe I'd work until I was 30, then that would be it. I was a product of the 50s and 60s. I thought I'd work up, and become famous pretty fast, like as a newspaper editor, and then I'd quit and get married and move to Westchester, have two children, and write novels, and live happily ever after.

4. *Most experienced a strong sense of visibility and heightened self-consciousness.*

Once inside the professions, the women met immediate challenges. Suddenly they realized that they definitely stood out within their offices. Their work environments had turned out to be far more male-dominated than were the universities where they had been trained. The women believed that because they were different, their performance was judged very closely. Many noted that their own high criteria for success grew even more extreme under these conditions.

5. *Subjects believed they were not taken seriously until they had proven their competence.*

These women were surprised to find out that many men were skeptical of their abilities. Most came to believe that the only way for a woman to gain credibility is by performing in an outstanding fashion. A financial analyst explained that this means a woman has to do better than her male peers in order to be seen as a professional equal.

> I think it's true with some people that you're going to meet that they do have this feeling that because you're a woman you are less competent, so you do need to prove yourself more. I certainly feel that way. I feel this great need to do very well. Certain people that you are working with, you sense that they are looking at you very closely and scrutinizing everything you do, and that if you are going to gain their respect and cooperation, you're going to have to be—maybe not 100% better than a man—but 150%.

An architect described how this same dynamic operates in the building industry.

> Out in the field I have to prove myself in the first half hour or I've lost it. That's because the contractors and the tradesmen don't expect you to know what you're doing. That can be a real problem. I think in the office it's true, too, because I have to fight harder for credibility with a client. You absolutely have to do that. I feel that I've really had to be more accommodating and I've had to work much harder at a design than have the guys. That's precisely because I'm fighting against these negative expectations. The odds are against you. You're guilty until proven innocent.

6. *Long hours and much hard work characterized the first few years.*

During this initial "testing" period most women did little else but work. As a result many felt that their personal relationships had become strained. Some women reported unexpected difficulties in their marriages and primary relationships, especially during the first two years of practice. Single women often worried that they did not have the time or energy necessary for meeting prospective partners. In a similar fashion many women noted that they missed spending time with good female friends.

In general an ease and impromptu quality had vanished from the women's personal lives. Many found that their peers had also become caught up in professional involvements, and that suddenly all social contact required complicated planning and advance scheduling. Over and over the women mentioned their lack of free time and their unmet wishes to take classes, to become active in their communities, to read, to relax, to see friends casually, "to live again."

Though most had gained a great deal of personal satisfaction from their careers, the majority were well aware of the sacrifices that success had required. Many wondered aloud whether what they had achieved had really been worth what they had given up.

As long as these women felt compelled to prove their ability in the office, however, most opted to work days and nights and weekends. Noting the skepticism among their male colleagues, many believed that their performance on the job had to be more than excellent—it had to be perfect. An architect described her feeling a sense of humiliation when she made even the slightest mistake.

> An average woman is not tolerated. You have to be exceptional. If I'm in an in-house critique and I'm asked a question for which I don't know the answer, I feel completely ashamed. I feel like I should have known, that I should always know that answer. Whereas for the men, they don't know all the answers and it just seems to roll off their backs. I feel as though I have to do a totally thorough job. I tell myself that that's not fair, but I still have this feeling, all the time.

7. *Becoming more assertive was valued but conflictual.*

Most women agreed that with time they had come to recognize the importance of being more assertive on the job. It is crucial to point out, however, that the question of assertiveness raised the most intense and clearly expressed conflicts for this group.

Specifically, when work required them to be openly aggressive and somewhat pushy, many individuals feared that they would lose their femininity. Though most found themselves having to adopt more assertive behaviors in order to be effective, a large number secretly felt uncomfortable and anxious. Torn between the real demands of their present professional roles and long-standing internalized notions about the correct female role, many experienced real confusion and fear. Several were worried that they had already begun to lose the more sensitive, gentle aspects of their personalities. Some wondered aloud whether they had even started to "turn into men."

On this issue the bankers, architects, and lawyers resembled other high-achieving females described in the literature. During the past decade a good deal of research has indicated that a perceived conflict between femininity and assertiveness is widespread among American working women (Horner, 1972; Bardwick, 1979; Rohrbaugh, 1979; Rohrlich, 1980). Many authors have noted that today's young professionals were raised with traditional values and sex-role stereotypes. All of a sudden, however, these same women find themselves thrust into a fast-paced, competitive work world. Psychologists have observed that during this period of rapid social change many female professionals feel pulled in both directions. They are caught between strong wishes for success and deep underlying wishes to maintain certain portions of a very traditional feminine role. When women feel anxious about their assertive behavior this fundamental conflict is being activated.

In analyzing her own experience, an attorney suggested that men may not suffer these same anxieties about assertiveness because they may not equate it with the potential loss of relationship. This woman recalled how her socialization had condemned aggressive behavior and had instead trained her to be "nice."

> In most situations my opposing counsel is a man and I want him to like me. That's contrary to the way you are supposed to work here. Whether he likes me or not should not be an issue at all. I think that because aggressiveness is tolerated and encouraged in men, they're used to it. They're expected to do it, so most of them don't feel uncomfortable. The whole thing of "being liked" is just not an issue for men. I remember as a kid

if I came home and said, "So-and-so doesn't like me," rather than say "Screw her!" or "Screw him!" or "So what?" my mother would say, "Now, tomorrow, you go in and tell this person that they look very good or that they've done something very well. Give them a compliment. Then that person will like you." I was never really allowed to have anyone dislike me. No wonder this is so hard.

8. *Women were starting to question the central role of work within their lives.*

Only after they had proven their competence to themselves and their colleagues did these women begin to doubt their career commitments. It was as if a certain measure of success in the work world had been required before most could stop and really think about the choices they had made. When they did, a good number of women recognized that they were very unsure about their professional futures. There were two primary reasons why this re-evaluation occurred with the intensity it did.

In the first place, many women had recently grown aware of the emotional and physical toll their professions had taken. Some told of bouts with illness while others recounted periods of profound depression. Mindful of the sacrifices they had been making, the majority expressed great interest in learning more about what they termed "stress."

Perhaps more significantly, however, women were uncertain about the future because they had grown increasingly critical of the cultural norms dictating behavior in most work environments. Specifically, women in this study had begun to question what they viewed as the excessively competitive work style common among professionals. Having taken a closer look at their own male-dominated organizations, many individuals were disenchanted with the life-styles and value systems they saw expressed. While working each day in rigid, hierarchical systems, some women fantasized about more flexible and collaborative organizations. A number were seriously considering becoming entrepreneurs or finding jobs in smaller more decentralized institutions.

The following words of a district attorney summarize the conflict that most women were just beginning to express.

Recently I have started to become tired. I've gone through so many different facets of self-questioning. The truth is that I'm still not really sure how to visualize myself in the role of a professional woman. It's two-edged because this experience has given me a great deal of confidence. A lot of positive things have happened. But on the other side, I don't know that I would be so serious if I weren't a lawyer. I have to portray a certain role and keep up a certain personality. But sometimes I'm not sure I want to be that person. I have fallen into a situation where my job has become very, very important. I put a lot of time and emotional energy into it. That's a bigger area of self-questioning, really. I keep wondering how it is that my job has become so important. Why I am living a life this way rather than in a different way?

In reviewing the central findings of this study it is clear that changing patterns of employment have created a host of new challenges for female professionals. In short the work place has become a psychologically loaded environment for men and women alike. Though the professions have undergone a tremendous amount of internal change, as yet there are no clear-cut norms. The resulting environment can be filled with great ambiguity and anxiety for all participants. To date most of that anxiety has been publicly denied.

IMPLICATIONS FOR CLINICAL PRACTICE

Given the findings of this research, what can therapists do to help young career women? I believe that the first thing clinicians need to understand is that most of these individuals are high-functioning adults who are facing new and unexpected demands. The women I talked to are strong people who are now somewhat bewildered over issues related to work and to adult life in general. Though they show little fear of success, these women do worry about retaining a sense of femininity while striving for high achievement. Many feel isolated at work. They feel cut off from one another and from sources of professional help.

In working with these women, psychotherapists need to keep in mind several key issues. First, clinicians can support young professional women by acknowledging that today many are being called upon to develop new and more assertive personal styles. Second, therapists can understand that there are important differences across the professions and that different psychological issues will develop depending upon the specific tasks that each woman is asked to perform. Third, psychotherapists can help women recognize that they are not unique in the problems they face working within male-dominated fields. While it is certainly true that individuals will bring different levels of conflict to each of these issues, for many professionals uncovering psychotherapy may not be indicated. A banking executive expressed her reluctance about entering into traditional therapy because she feared that her concerns about work life would be overlooked. This woman drew a powerful analogy between her daily battles and those of a soldier in Vietnam.

> My chief complaint against most clinicians is that they usually focus on doing lifework therapy instead of focusing on your immediate needs and your day-to-day life. It's like taking some guy and throwing him into Vietnam and then asking him how he was raised. Of course that's important, but somebody shooting at him on a day-by-day basis is what's really important today. And for a lot of women, we're being shot at every day in corporate America. That's what I'd like to deal with in therapy because I really need to.

Based upon these research findings I'd like to offer some specific suggestions for clinical practice. My first recommendation is that psychotherapists take the initiative and make the availability of their services far more visible to those inside the business world. Despite the obvious sophistication of the group I interviewed, these women were surprisingly uninformed about the variety of services offered within their communities. Clinicians need to go out to professional women where they live and work. If it is assumed that women who need treatment will always seek out a therapist, a large number of potential clients may never be reached.

Secondly, the psychotherapeutic community must create and offer new treatment modalities designed to address the specific needs of this population. One possibility is short-term therapy. Another is group work that would focus on the unique problems of one or two professional groups. A third idea is for more educationally-oriented events co-sponsored by clinicians and other professional women. Those with experience in a certain field could advise beginners, not on how to "dress for success," but on how to handle anxieties about performance.

History has demonstrated that women in this culture show great strength in being able to use friends and support groups effectively. Clinicians can surely rely on the resources of professional women to bring valuable new dimensions to the therapeutic process.

Throughout this work it is essential that therapists be sensitive to the kinds of emotional armor that many women in male-dominated fields have had to assume. The strains associated with a highly competitive and often ruthless business world have required certain women to adopt somewhat rigid defensive styles in order to survive. At the present time there may be a wide gap between the professional experiences of women psychotherapists and the types of women I interviewed. Differences in background, training, and daily work worlds may mean that at first there will be a need to build understanding between the groups. While clinicians may view certain business women as overly defended or non-introspective, it is possible that some professional women may see psychotherapists as having opted out of the "real world." Since these initial projections could interfere with the building of a critical therapeutic alliance, these issues must be discussed openly and early on in the process.

My own experience is that women in clinical practice and women working in male-dominated organizations can work together in an effective and dynamic fashion. As individuals each of us can acknowledge the presence of sex discrimination and bias within our culture. As women we need to underscore the common elements of our experience and to share together the professional expertise each has developed. These common bonds need to be clarified and accentuated in the services clinicians can offer to beginning professional women.

REFERENCES

Bardwick, J. M. *In Transition*. New York: Holt, Rinehart and Winston, 1979.

Epstein, C. W. *Woman's Place*. Berkeley: University of California Press, 1970.

Epstein, C. W. *Women in Law*. New York: Basic Books, Inc., 1981.

Harragan, B. L. *Games Mother Never Taught You*. New York: Warner Books, 1977.

Hennig, M. and Jardim, A. *The Managerial Woman*. New York: Pocket Books, 1976.

Horner, M. S. The Motive to Avoid Success and Changing Aspirations of College Women. In J. M. Bardwick (Ed.), *Readings on the Psychology of Women*. New York: Harper and Row, 1972.

Kanter, R. M. *Men and Women of the Corporation*. New York: Basic Books, 1977.

Laws, J. L. The Psychology of Tokenism: an Analysis. *Sex Roles: A Journal of Research*, 1975, 1 (1), 51-67.

Rohrbaugh, J. B. *Women: Psychology's Puzzle*. New York: Basic Books, 1979.

Rohrlich, J. B. *Work and Love: The Crucial Balance*. New York: Summit Books, 1980.

Rossi, A. S. Barriers to Career Choice of Engineering, Medicine, or Science among American Women. In J. A. Mattfeld and C. G. Aken (Eds.), *Women and the Scientific Professions*. Cambridge: Massachusetts Institute of Technology Press, 1965.

Standley, K., and Soules, B. Women in Male-Dominated Professions: Contrasts in their Personal and Vocational Histories. *Journal of Vocational Behavior*, 1974, *4* (2), 245-258.

Tangri, S. S. Determinants of Occupational Role Innovation Among College Women. *Journal of Social Issues*, 1972, *28*, 177-199.

Trigg, L. J. and Perlman, D. Social Influences on Women's Pursuit of a Non-Traditional Career. *Psychology of Women Quarterly*, 1976, *11*, 1-18.

The Consequences
of Abortion Legislation

Marjorie Braude

Every major stage in the revolution taking place in the rights of women has produced its counter revolution which would limit or remove its gains. Twentieth century United States has produced a two-stage revolution in favor of women's reproductive freedom. The first stage is the development, legalization, spread of information and utilization of contraception. The second is the legalization of abortion which occurred primarily through the Supreme Court in the *Roe vs. Wade* decision in 1973. This paper examines some of the factual consequences of that decision and the prospective consequences of some of the legislation proposed at this time with intent to reverse or nullify the effects of the decision. It examines relevant research information concerning pregnancy and abortion which make clearer some of the consequences of variations in government policies upon the lives of women, children and families.

First, let us take a look at some of the philosophical assumptions which underlie the debate about reproductive rights. On the one hand is the assumption that the decision whether or not to carry a baby to term is an individual decision, as part of the individual rights guaranteed by the Constitution. Further, since it is the woman who carries, delivers, and usually nurtures the baby, it is her decision to make over her own body and life. Another major assumption is that responsible and voluntary decision making on the part of individuals is desirable for the responsible conceiving and raising of children. Also, the maximum health and safety of mother and child is held to be a primary value. For those of us who proceed from these assumptions, *Roe vs. Wade* has brought immense progress.

The author is a psychiatrist in private practice and on the staff of Westwood Hospital. She is treasurer of the American Medical Women's Association, Women's Committee Southern California Psychiatric Society. She was co-moderator, Women's Institutes, American Ortho-Psychiatric Association, 1982 and 1983.

On the other hand, we have those whose religious and/or political beliefs are that the decision to complete a pregnancy must be controlled by the state, and that individual freedom to make this decision is a license for irresponsible sex and life styles. Central to this view is a radical shift in our traditional way of viewing life and personhood as starting with birth or with breath (Genesis 2:7). The new moralists would have us consider life as dating from the moment when egg and sperm join to become the beginning of an embryo. They consider an embryo from this moment not as a prospective life or a life in formation but as an unborn child or person. They wish to legalize this by adding a "human life" amendment to the United States Constitution which would state this principle, and in its most powerful form give the fetus a legal entity and rights to survival paramount over those of its mother. Associated with this is a series of attempts to change our legal and social practices regarding fetuses to consider them as persons. This includes such things as giving them the right to sue and treating dead fetuses as dead persons instead of surgical specimens by giving them funerals, ceremonial burials, and autopsies (Braude, 1982).

Biologically a substantial number of fetuses spontaneously die and abort. Many fertilized eggs do not successfully implant in the wall of the uterus and die. Some spontaneously die or abort after implantation, of which some are defectively formed.

Socially, the decision to keep or terminate a pregnancy is not made in isolation. Sex and pregnancy can be voluntary or involuntary actions. A pregnancy can have an enormous range of consequences in the life of a woman. It can make her a social success by providing a desired child and heir, or it can result in the loss of her family and social status, loss of educational and job opportunity, and complete social ostracism, depending upon her circumstances and the social views and actions of those who have power over her life (Petchesky, 1980).

Historically, abortion has always taken place. The variables have been, 1) who is empowered to make the decision about it and, 2) the safety and technology of the procedure. At times women have had the right to make the decision, or the right to make it under some circumstances, such as prior to the sensation of fetal movement which is known as quickening. Prior to modern techniques of ascertaining pregnancy, quickening was considered the beginning of life. More often the legal decision has been made by church or state (Mohr, 1978). It was illegal in twentieth century United States until laws began to change in the late 1960s, climaxed in 1973 when the Supreme Court in *Roe vs. Wade* decreed that abortion was a part of a woman's right to privacy. This does not make abortion specifically guaranteed under the Constitution. This brought about a revolution in the availability of abortion services for some of us. At the same time those who oppose this decision, particularly the Roman Catholic and Mormon Churches, have powerfully organized their opposition. Since hospitals are largely sponsored by religious groups, no Roman Catholic hospitals and only 31% of non-Catholic hospitals provided any abortion services in 1977. This has given rise to independent abortion clinics, predominantly in urban areas (Jaffe, 1981).

Eight years of legal abortion have produced a public health revolution in both maternal and child health. In 1965 when abortion was illegal, 235 or 20% of deaths which were reported as related to pregnancy and childbirth were due to abortion. Since abortions were concealed this probably represents an under reporting. This number has dropped steadily with relaxation of abortion laws to 45 deaths in 1973, and 18 deaths in 1977. In New York and California during the 1960s, almost 20% of pregnancy-related admissions to municipal hospitals were related to illegal abortions. In California the number of hospital admissions for an infected uterus following an illegal abortion sharply declined with the first availability of legal abortion. They declined from 69 per 1000 live births in 1967 to 22 per 1000 live births in 1979, the year after the passage of a therapeutic abortion law (Stewart, 1971).

The risk of dying from a term pregnancy is seven times that of dying from an abortion. In addition 10 to 15% of term pregnancies are delivered by Caesarean section which present the mother with risks of major surgery. The risk of having to undergo major surgery for a complication of legal abortion is approximately one one-hundreth of that of carrying a pregnancy to term (Cates, 1982).

The survival and health of the infant has also improved. One study done at Harlem Hospital in New York showed a decrease of infant mortality from 33.0 per 1000 live births in 1969 to 18.9 deaths in 1971, largely due to a decreased number of low birth weight babies (Glass, 1974).

This improvement is despite the fact that legal abortion has never become fully available, especially to poor, rural, minority and teenage women. Of the 23% of counties that have services, most of them are urban, requiring women to travel. In 1978 although 1.4 million women had legal abortions an estimated 479,000 women, identified primarily as minority and low income women, were unable to obtain desired abortions. We do not have an accurate way of knowing the number of abortions prior to legalization since statistics were not kept. Estimates range from 200,000 to 2,000,000 in the 1960s (Cates, 1982).

While the medical profession and hospitals have been slow to take leadership in establishing abortion facilities, legislators have been very active in limiting abortion by large numbers of detailed restrictions. They restrict funding, especially for poor women, establish physical standards for abortion facilities, waiting periods, permission and special reporting requirements.

The public health gains can be reversed. In Eastern European countries abortion was liberalized during the 1950s and later made illegal when their government became concerned about a declining birth rate. In Rumania the number of deaths from abortion more than doubled in the year following the enactment of the restrictive birth law (Djerassi, 1979). So far the partial reversal of abortion funding due to restrictions on public funding or other restrictions on how and where abortions can be performed has produced a slight increase in mortality but not this dramatic reversal. Whether this is because these women have simply carried their pregnancies to term or whether the women were able to find other resources and pay for them, or because the modern suction technique for early abortion is relatively non-invasive and easy for an amateur to perform, is not clear.

A detailed study has been done on those women who died from abortions between 1975 and 1979. They were older than women who sought legal abortions and disproportionately Black and Hispanic. Over half induced the abortion themselves, then died primarily from infection or air embolism. They used instillation of cleaning solutions, catheters or other objects. Financial considerations and a desire to keep the abortion secret were the most frequent motivations (Binken, Gold, & Cates, 1982).

There has been a great deal of research checking out possible adverse psychological effects on the mother. The largest was done in Britain by Colin Brewer (1977) who studied the incidence of psychosis following abortion and childbirth in a population of over one million people in a fifteen month period. There was one report of psychosis following abortion in a woman who had two prior psychoses following childbirth. There are many other studies which show abortion to be felt as transient loss which is responded to by the mother as any other loss with few adverse consequences. Sometimes there are positive emotional consequences because a problem has been solved (Brody, 1971).

Physically abortion is quite safe and the earlier it is performed the safer it is. Each year since 1973 women have been obtaining abortions earlier in pregnancy. In 1973, less than 40% of women obtained them before nine weeks of pregnancy. By 1978, over half were obtained before nine weeks and over nine in ten were obtained in the first twelve weeks, or during the first trimester. In 1978, less than one percent were obtained after twenty weeks. This is despite the fact that there are serious complications of pregnancy such as high blood pressure which do not arise until late pregnancy. Also, amniocentesis to determine if a woman is carrying a fetus afflicted with a severe genetic disorder cannot be performed until the middle of the second trimester (Guttmacher Institute, 1982). Since there is a great concern on the part of abortion opponents about abortions performed late in pregnancy on possibly viable infants, this low incidence of abortions after twenty weeks is of interest.

A major prospective study was carried out at Kaiser Hospital in San Francisco. They interviewed 8,000 women from 1959 to 1967 when abortion was still illegal who received prenatal care through the Kaiser Health Plan. They asked them early in their pregnancy, "How do you feel about having a baby now?" The responses were categorized as strongly favorable, ambivalent or negative. The pregnancy and birth histories of these women and their babies were then studied for a number of factors. Some of them were markedly different for women who did not want their pregnancies. Perinatal death* was approximately double in those women who did not want their pregnancies, and severe congenital anomalies, postpartum infection and hemorrhage, anxiety states, and accidental injuries during pregnancy were all much higher in the unwanted group. The proportion of women who required three doses or more of medication for pain during labor were also significantly higher. The increase of accidental injuries during pregnancy was considered to be related to stress (Laukaran, 1980).

Two European studies followed out the lives of the children of mothers who were refused abortion as compared with carefully selected control groups. Forssman and Thuwe (1971) in Sweden

---

*Death of the fetus within four weeks after birth.

followed 120 children of such mothers until they were 21 years old. They had over twice as many indices of insecure childhood such as illegitimacy, foster home placement, complaints to authorities, and death or divorce of a parent. They had almost twice as many reports of crime or delinquency, educational inadequacy and need for psychiatric help. A Czechoslovakian study on a similar group in which 220 children were followed for nine years showed similar increased indices of family instability and problems of "maladaptation" on the part of children, particularly the boys (Matijcik, 1978).

Another prospective study performed on 32 normal married women in the third trimester of pregnancy shows acceptance of pregnancy had an effect upon labor. Women who did not accept their pregnancy had longer labors and more anxiety (Lederman, 1981).

The United States has one of the highest teenage pregnancy rates in the developed world. About 40% of the women in their teens become pregnant and about 20% give birth at least once. In 1978, out of 1,142,000 pregnancies of women under 20, 38% ended in abortion, 22% resulted in births to unmarried mothers, 17% were born to married mothers, 10% were born to mothers who married subsequent to becoming pregnant, and 13% miscarried. All of the problem indices are higher. Premature birth, perinatal loss and complications of labor and delivery are more frequent, particularly in the younger adolescent.

Although most births to unmarried mothers are unintended, 87% of unmarried teenage mothers keep their children. The price that is paid by the mother is in cutting short her education, having less job opportunity and lower income. The children have lower IQ and achievement scores than others and are more likely to repeat grades (Guttmacher Institute, 1981).

Rape is an increasingly common event. Some women who are raped become pregnant. In addition to the other factors affecting an unwanted pregnancy, the rape victim has to deal with the profound psychological consequences of having violence inflicted upon the intimate parts of her body. The consequences are severe and often last for years. The pregnancy is felt and known by the mother to be the seed of violence. To force the victim of assault to bear the pregnancy is to further violate her person and to force her to feel the effects of violence which inevitably has profound effects upon the child.

The American Humane Association did a detailed analysis of 250 reported sex crimes against persons age sixteen or under sixteen in 1969. These included both rape and incest. Nine out of ten victims were female and the pregnancy rate was twelve percent (DeFrancis, 1969).

Incest is not uncommon and becoming increasingly documented. Pregnancy rates in incest, when documented, are higher than rape, possibly because of multiple exposures. It is frequently a multi-generational phenomenon which is profoundly disruptive to families. The pregnancy which results disrupts the life of the mother on every level. The situation of a 12-year-old girl who gives birth to her father's child is profoundly disruptive. Probable secrets are revealed with consequences that may break up the family. The girl is profoundly alienated from the experiences of school and peers (Meiselman, 1979). The child born of such a pregnancy is at risk to become yet another victim of sexual or physical abuse and to carry the pattern on to the next generation.

Another group that would have no recourse are women who have amniocentesis and discover that their baby will be born defective. Older women with a greater risk of congenitally defective children may then not risk having a child so for them a denial of abortion will also be a denial of childbirth.

The proposed Human Life Amendment to the Constitution would make abortion a capital crime which would place the mother and others involved in legal jeopardy as murderers. It would bring government into each bedroom since one's private conduct during pregnancy and the causes of any miscarriage could be subjects of investigation. By conferring legal personhood upon the fetus it would acquire full rights, including the right to sue and pay taxes. Who would have the right to sue on behalf of the fetus? Could a fetus sue a mother who smokes during pregnancy? Could government stop a woman from taking medication, or working at her job if there were any possible risk to the pregnancy? Since one does not know the moment of conception in advance, could women of childbearing age be limited from jobs because of hazard to a possible pregnancy? Would methods of birth control which prevent implantation of the fertilized egg such as the IUD be banned? How much of contraceptive research would be outlawed? These are some of the consequences to be considered and questions to be answered.

Some within the anti-abortion movement make an attempt to justify their position as scientific rather than philosophic. One attempt is made by Dr. Bernard Nathanson, a gynecologist. He defines the implanted fetus as alive because it has unique genetic characteristics and distinguishable biochemical reactions. He equates the beginnings of heartbeat, brainwaves, and the shapes of organs in the fetus with life. Following this logic he feels that the deaths of a few hundred mothers from illegal abortions are permissible when equated against the deaths of a million fetuses. He also finds the birth of a child who is the product of rape or incest acceptable, and would accept abortion only where the life of the mother is directly threatened. His hope for a resolution of the dilemma lies in advancing technology which will some day permit a fetus to be removed and to develop in another life support system if the mother cannot or will not do so (Nathanson, 1979).

Those who consider the life of the fetus paramount have joined in organizations which have a Messianic zeal toward saving the lives of the unborn. They practice "non-violent direct action" against abortion clinics, which includes many kinds of harassment against clinics and the persons coming to them for services.

In Chicago an anti-abortion group went to great lengths to prevent an eleven-year-old girl from having an abortion. They hired a detective to find her mother, went unannounced to her home and used stratagems to contact her after she refused to see them, and picketed the hospital where they thought the abortion was taking place (Plain Dealer, 1982). The anti-abortion group obviously did not consider the privacy and the freedom of action of the family as values, nor did they appear to show concern for the impact of this pregnancy on the quality of life of the eleven-year-old or the fetus should it become born. The medical tradition of privacy and confidentiality of the doctor-patient relationship is clearly being challenged by such actions.

Political and social policy is frequently backed up or justified by what are considered to be relevant medical and scientific facts. For this reason inaccurate information needs to be corrected. For example, the right-to-life organization sponsored a full-page newspaper advertisement with a picture of a live infant and a text which stated that 160,000 abortions are performed in the fifth, sixth, and seventh month of pregnancy (Los Angeles Times, 1980). The federal Center for Disease Control was given as the source of the figures. When asked, they stated the number to be between ten and thirteen thousand, so the figure in the advertisement was a gross overstatement.

We have a large body of information supporting the physical, psychological and social benefits of legal abortion to women, children and families. We also have information that adverse psychological consequences are minimal. We have a division of our society into two camps. On the one hand we have those who appreciate the benefits described and support woman's right to make decisions about her own body. On the other hand we have those who are religiously and philosophically opposed because they define life to include the fetus, and therefore the protection of that life becomes paramount over almost all other considerations to mother, child and family.

All of us would prefer to see fewer abortions. Most of us want to see the decrease come from better education and contraceptive methods rather than coercion. We would like to see our respect for individual rights fully include the right of a woman to make free and informed decisions over her own body and future. It is the woman who experiences the responsibility and hazards of bringing life into the world, and it is she who has the most information about whether she, hopefully with the help of the child's father and others, can properly support that life.

REFERENCES

Braude, M., Lang, D., Lang, J., & Olsen W. Myths and assumptions of antiabortionists. *Journal of American Medical Women's Association,* March, 1982, *Vol. 3,* 74-76.

Brewer, C. Incidence of post abortion psychosis: a prospective study. *British Medical Journal,* February 1977, *Vol. 1,* 476-477.

Brody, M., Meikle, E., & Gerritse, R. Therapeutic abortion: a prospective study. *American Journal of Obstetrics and Gynecology,* February 1, 1971, *Vol. 109,* No. 3, 347-353.

Cates, W. Legal abortion: the public health record. *Science,* March 26, 1982, *Vol. 215,* No. 4540, 1586-1590.

Center for Disease Control. *Abortion surveillance; annual summary 1977.* Center for Disease Control, Family Planning Division, Atlanta, Georgia 30333, September 1979.

De Francis, V. *Protecting the child victim of sex crimes committed by adults; Brooklyn-Bronx study.* Denver, Colorado: American Humane Association, 1969.

Djerassi, C. *The politics of contraception.* New York: W. W. Norton, 1979.

Forssman, H., & Thuwe, I. One hundred and twenty children born after application for therapeutic abortion refused. *ACTA Psychiatrica Scandinavia,* 1971, Vol. 42, 71-88.

Genesis. "And the Lord God formed man of the dust of the ground, and breathed into his nostrils the breath of life: and man became a living soul." *Holy Bible,* King James Version, Chapter 2, verse 7.

Glass, L., Evans, H., Swartz, D., Rajegowda, B. L. K., & Leblanc, W. Effects of legalized abortion on neonatal mortality and obstetrical morbidity at Harlem Hospital Center. *American Journal of Public Health,* July, 1974, *Vol 64,* No 7, 717-718.

Guttmacher Institute. Abortion and public health: the facts. *Issue in Brief,* October 1981, *Vol 1,* No. 9. 1220 19th St., N.W., Washington, D. C. 20036.

Guttmacher Institute. *Teenage Pregnancy: the problem that hasn't gone away.* 1981. 360 Park Avenue South, New York, N. Y. 10010.

Jaffe, F., Lef, P., & Lindheim, B. *Abortion politics; private Morality and public policy.* New York: McGraw-Hill Book Company, 1981.

Laukaran, V., & van den Berg, B. The relationship of maternal attitude to pregnancy outcomes and obstetric complications. *American Journal of Obstetrics and Gynecology,* February 1, 1980, *Vol 136,* No. 3, 374-379.

Lederman, R., Lederman, E., Work, A., & McCann, D. Relationship of psychological factors in pregnancy to progress in labor. *Nursing Research,* March-April 1979, *Vol. 28,* No. 2, 94-97.

Matijcik, Z., Dytrych, Z., & Schuller, V. Children from unwanted pregnancies, *ACTA Psychiatrica Scandinavia,* 1978, *Vol. 57,* No. 1, 67-90.

Meiselman, K. *Incest.* Jossey-Bass, 1979.

Mohr, J. *Abortion in America.* New York: Oxford University Press, 1978.

Mother is firm on child's abortion. *Plain Dealer,* Cleveland, Ohio: June 10, 1982.

Petchesky, R. P. Reproductive freedom: beyond "a woman's right to choose." *Signs,* Summer 1980, *Vol 5,* No. 4, 661-685.

Right to Life League. Advertisement. *Los Angeles Times,* Los Angeles: July 31, 1980, 24.

Stewart, G., & Goldstein, P. Therapeutic abortion in California. *Obstetrics and Gynecology,* April, 1971, *Vol 37,* No. 4, 510-514.

VALUING OUR SELVES

This section is a celebration of the many faces and voices of woman. It is written by and about women who have felt the double or multiple oppression of being female in a male centered society, and not fitting into the cultural stereotype of the "All American Girl." By that limited standard, a woman is made to feel invisible, unloved and worthless unless she is young, blond, blue-eyed, thin, middle-class, heterosexual, beautiful, and always smiling. Like all of us, the women in these pages deviate from this artificial norm in more ways than one. We all share what Adrienne Rich (1979) calls "the intersection of oppression and strength, damage and beauty."*

The themes of conflict and wholeness, of healing the double bind, reemerge in this section as they apply to the particular circumstances of women of color, women who are lesbian, Jewish, middle-aged. Devalued and pathologized by psychology and society, these women express for all of us the urgent need to recover our own strength and dignity. We begin by trusting and valuing our own definitions of self, the effectiveness of our successful coping patterns, and rejecting the definitions imposed by those who do not share our values or our history. The introductory poem sets the stage for each woman to find her own way out of the crippling and rigid patterns imposed by the patriarchy.

These distinct and separate voices of women harmonize in a chorus more powerful than any voice alone, far richer and more complex than any single melody or single standard or normality. Together, these voices have the potential to influence our understanding of *all women,* and to challenge the practice of therapy. We learn to acknowledge our differences, the complexity of each individual woman and discard the stereotypes that keep us from accepting ourselves and each other.

---

*Rich, A. Power and danger: works of a common woman, in *On lies, secrets, and silence*, New York: W. W. Norton & Co., 1979.

In these papers we remind therapists to return to an earlier tradition that focused on listening and learning from the client's own truth. Feminist therapy reaffirms that perspective. We search for truth in the client's own words and feelings. We believe her pain and resist defining her by standards other than her own. We find her strength and build on it.

Message from Antarctica

I've started back now.
Had you given me up for lost?
Frostbitten, nearly snowblind,
Sick of penguins in tuxedo straightjackets
   squabbling like chickens,
I'm heading north (which way is up?)
It'll take a while.
Wait for me.

Anonymous

A Message from Antarctica is the first poem of a middle-aged woman in therapy.

Change and Creativity at Midlife

Rachel Josefowitz Siegel

At 58, I am enjoying what Margaret Mead called PMZ, post-menopausal-zest. I look back at my midlife years as a period of sometimes painful, sometimes exhilarating change, growth, and creativity. I look ahead at the next decade and wonder what it will be like.

My turning point into midlife came with a frightening jolt when my husband suffered and survived a sudden heart attack. He was 47, I was 39. This sudden awareness of death became an organizing force for me. Life assumed an urgency and an intensity which were at first nearly paralyzing and gradually became liberating.

At 44, I suffered another shock to my system, when my gynecologist insisted on removing my uterus. I experienced this physical and symbolic invasion of my inner being, my sexual self, as a loss of youth, of femininity, of my place and function in the world. These feelings were deeply rooted and transmitted through my female ancestors, generations of Eastern European Jewish mothers, for whom the act of giving birth gave the only acceptable meaning to their lives, constituting their personal contribution to the survival of a severely oppressed and persecuted people. These feelings were also nurtured and reinforced by the American culture to which I was transplanted in my teens. In this new world the beauty contest still set the standard for female worth and accomplishment; the bust, waist, and hip measurements of movie stars and airline hostesses were of public interest, and the feminine mystique was in full swing.

The year of my operation was also the year my daughter and youngest child left for college and my two sons were called up for the Vietnam war. When they were both rejected because of allergies

The author is a feminist therapist in private practice in Ithaca, New York, and co-editor of this book. She was co-moderator of the Women's Institute, American Orthopsychiatric Association, 1981 & 1982.

An earlier version of this paper appeared as "A midlife journey from housewife to psychotherapist," in *Voices: the Art and Science of Psychotherapy*, Spring 1982, *18*, 1, 29-33.

and flat feet, my relief was nearly as great as my anxiety had been. The accumulation of midlife separations, losses and near-losses left me with a profound sense of powerlessness.

To say that I was depressed during those years, or that my world had fallen apart would be simplistic. I continued to function. I had been a full-time homemaker and community volunteer. I now became director of our religious school. Looking back, it does not surprise me that my activities focused on Jewish children at that time as a way of continuing my traditional role.

Long ago I had dreamed of medical school, of becoming a psychoanalyst. No one had taken me seriously and neither had I. Like many women of my generation, I gave up the dream. I married young and acted as if this dream replaced the other; I made a career of homemaking and mothering. The end of this career felt like the end of my life.

Every afternoon around four or five o'clock, no matter how busy I had been or how much I had accomplished, I would feel an immense lassitude, a sadness, a sense of utter futility and uselessness. Another empty day gone by, for I discounted all my activities. They did not have the recognition or the rewards of paid work or the legitimacy of a profession, nor did they challenge my full potential. And then another evening alone with my husband, just the two of us, he immersed in his work, at the peak of his career and somewhat distant, and both of us uncomfortable with the potential for greater intimacy.

A return to therapy only increased my sense of useless dependency, for neither the therapist nor I knew enough to relate my discomfort to the realities of a middle-aged housewife facing the rest of her life without an acceptable role. He wanted to focus on early psychosexual content, which we did over and over again. Therapy became one more experience in which my present concerns and activities were discounted and made invisible. The guilt and dependency were reinforced. The message was: if I stopped resisting and acting out, the neurosis could be cured and I would no longer be so unnecessarily depressed. I got through this difficult period, gradually replacing the midlife mourning with midlife planning, shifting my energies from the past to the future. One day my daughter gave me a poster that said "Today is the first day of the rest of your life." I was ready to move: I applied to graduate school.

I entered the social-work program at Syracuse University, commuting 60 miles to classes. The learning process was both painful and exhilarating. I traded in my familiar faculty-wife, homemaker status for the risk of testing myself and exposing my ignorance in new situations. I rediscovered my brain and my sense of competence in the world.

I immersed myself in the writings of Karen Horney (1967), Thomas Szasz (1961, 1965), and R. D. Laing (1950), exploring the arbitrary and elusive quality of concepts of mental illness and mental health, and their relationship to socio-economic factors and to power relationships. I was excited by the process of sorting out ideas about the self in society, and learning to understand myself and my clients more fully.

The emotional learning through my interactions with clients was profound, unsettling, and rewarding. Now on the other side of the therapy experience, I saw other women and tuned in to their pain. Many had not had the advantages of education, a comfortable middle-class environment, and a loving nonviolent husband which had been mine to take for granted. I became aware of my privileged position and of the oppression of women in our society. I began to question the male-centered and male-dominant structures of our society and the male definitions of women's experiences.

Becoming a therapist and a feminist was a complicated and confusing process. The inner turmoil was no longer without a purpose, yet still distressing, leading me once again to more personal therapy. This time I had a better idea of what I wanted from the therapeutic experience. I was a year or two ahead of other middle-aged women returning to school and was feeling very isolated and a little crazy for putting myself through such an ordeal. I looked for a therapist who would understand that my involvement in a new career was worth the difficulties and adjustments in family relationships that ensued. I was not ready to trust a woman, afraid she might be as confused and conflicted about these issues as I was. I chose an analyst whose wife was a prominent, outspoken professional woman, hoping that living with her would qualify him to understand me. The fact that he was Jewish seemed irrelevant but soon felt important. It was a good choice.

This time the therapy included all aspects of my life. I began to feel recognized and validated in all my complexity as a person with a past, a present and a future. We explored and legitimized my dreams of autonomous selfhood, the envy and ambition that were so closely tied to each other, the sense of urgency that permeates every midlife transition, the fears of aging, of living alone, and of sudden death that translated into a fear of living. I came to understand that I had suffered what Robert Seidenberg (1973) calls the "trauma of eventlessness." Later yet, when I read Jean Baker Miller (1976) I began to appreciate how difficult and complicated it is for a woman to shift from helping others grow to helping herself grow. I had chosen a profession in which I continued to help others grow and could do so only to the extent that I took my own growth as seriously as that of my clients.

As a beginning therapist, I became aware of and rejoiced in the spiraling loops of personal and professional development, each experience enriching the other. It is a process which I continue to appreciate, as my clients continue to teach me and I continue to make the therapy more meaningful with the accumulation of my own experiences.

My self-image changed as I gained confidence in my work. I heard clients talk about me as formidable, wise, calm, and understanding. I began to see myself as a person imbued with an authority I did not claim or wish to exercise, and a wisdom which I conveyed without fully trusting myself. I recognized the implied power of my position as a therapist, and the risk of misusing it. Fortunately, my sense of humor was also released as I became more sure of myself, and I began to use it as a therapeutic tool and to keep myself from falling into self-righteous pomposity. As my confidence grew, I continued to reach for new challenges.

By now, I was calling myself a feminist therapist, avidly reading the new literature by and about women: Jean Baker Miller (1973, 1975), Jessie Bernard (1972), Dorothy Dinnerstein (1977), Adrienne Rich (1977, 1979), Alexandra Kaplan (1976), and many others, exploring the possibility of non-sexist perspectives on the human condition and on therapy. By focusing fully on women's experiences I began to understand some of the broader social forces which keep both women and men locked into self-limiting roles and mutually destructive patterns.

It was lonely and frightening to be in disagreement with the established mainstream of my profession, to be questioning the values and practices of so many of my colleagues. I felt a need to interact with other women who were not afraid of feminism and who were intently exploring similar ideas. I began to attend conferences and to build a network of women who shared my interest and excitement in the emerging field of feminist therapy and womens' studies. At the annual meeting of the American Orthopsychiatric Association's Institute on Women, I found a supportive and stimulating forum for exchanging ideas and renewing my energy and enthusiasm. This validation of my feminist consciousness among my peers encouraged me to greater creativity. Again, with a leap into the risk-taking of self-exposure, now in the professional world of women colleagues, I became part of the planning collective for the Institute and presented my first paper (Siegel, 1982) at the Toronto meeting in 1980. There, for the first time, I also shared my idea for this book with the members of the collective, and found in Joan Hamerman Robbins a willing, imaginative and energetic ally, partner, collaborator and co-editor (see Introduction).

Back home, during the early years of private practice and agency work, I had seen many women who were physically and emotionally battered and whose needs were not met by community agencies. I became part of a study/consultation group which was part of the nucleus of a volunteer task force for battered women. We read Dell Martin (1976) and Lenore Walker (1979). We learned to recognize and to tolerate our own and our clients' feelings of rage, fear, depression, powerlessness, ambivalence, and learned helplessness, as we began to develop and improve direct services for battered women and to educate the community about these conditions. I felt a connection to these victims of male violence, having experienced the much less physically coercive but very real psychological battering of all women in our society. I also found a profound connection between the plight of battered women and the insecurities and powerlessness of my own childhood as a wandering Jew in the Europe of the Hitler years. There too the danger had been acute, the available options for escape had been limited and had meant giving up all that was familiar. The reality had been denied by a society which colluded with the perpetrator of violence by turning its back on and blaming the victims.

In the natural progression of my work with women and women's issues and my questioning of age and sex roles, the centrality of our culture's "heterosexual imperative" (Rich, 1980) became apparent to me. Adrienne Rich's concept opened a world of new perceptions about sexual choices, lesbian and heterosexual life-styles and the politics of patriarchy. My work with lesbian clients grew and my interactions with lesbian colleagues and friends were enriched as I opened myself to the possibility of reevaluating and understanding my own sexual and affectional choices, attractions and inhibitions from this new perspective.

I enjoyed this period of professional growth and stimulation within the context of other midlife changes. Among these were the hot flashes of menopause, confusing and disconcerting until I figured out what they were. My gynecologist and internist were equally unhelpful, assuming that I was asking for medication, when I was looking for information and a confirmation of my own observations. It was a great relief to talk with other women, to demystify and demedicalize this natural process. We who are no longer young enough to procreate, helped each other create new ways of valuing our bodies and our individual experiences of the later years of life. We shared a sense of discovery in observing our own body rhythms and occasional discomforts, and a sense of wonder at the wide range of individual physiological and emotional patterns. The value of our sharing led to a collaboration with Mickey Goldstein, a long-time friend and colleague, in planning and co-leading menopause workshops for other women.

The themes which continue to emerge in my clinical and educational work with women invariably interact with inner currents of my past and present life. The one stimulates the other. Sometimes the connection is obvious as in the menopause workshops and midlife presentations; sometimes it is more puzzling and obscure. The focus on victims of violence and the more recent interest in the lesbian experience have evoked personal memories and feelings of combined female and Jewish victimization and otherness. The victim blaming, the ambivalence of allegiance and identity, the self-devaluation are experienced by the members of any devalued and subordinate class or group in society.

As a Jew and as a woman I am an outsider, as a Jew and a woman I continue to confront the double task of coping with external oppression and discrimination, and sorting out the internal conflicts of being Jewish and being a woman. What kind of Jew? What kind of Woman? The answers keep shifting, the questions get deeper and the process more complex and colorful. The connections are as profound as the contradictions. Jewish sexism and heterosexism and feminist antisemitism are equally painful to me. My Jewish reality is often invisible among women, and my feminist reality is equally invisible among Jews. These areas of invisibility and contradiction have presented hurdles to my creativity in the form of fear—fear of being visible, misunderstood, open to rejection, criticism, disapproval and derision. Paradoxically, they also constitute the very challenge to creativity that motivates me to self-expression. The fear is overcome in the act of becoming visible, of being heard, of using language to communicate. As the skills of communication improve with each experience, the courage grows to try again. Essential to confronting my own fears has been a suppportive network of feminist friends, colleagues and family.

Throughout these midlife transitions and challenges, I have puzzled over and been fascinated by the interactions of physiological aging and the changes in role, in family composition, in sense of self in the world and how these differ for women and for men. I have tried to sort out the cultural and the biological, the personal and the political, coming to a deeper understanding of the ways in which they are all enmeshed. This has helped me in my work with people of all ages.

I no longer think of myself as a beginner in my career. The external process of balancing work, self and family without playing superwoman is still a challenge. The internal process of mutually enriching my work, my self and my family continues to be a joy. The man I married 38 years ago continues to confront his own aging body and enjoy his own work much as I do. Our marriage has weathered many storms, becoming more interesting and more fun. The recurring emotional theme in my life is no longer that of eventlessness, loss, and emptiness, but rather richness, occasional overload, and stimulation. There is not enough time or energy to do all that I wish to do. I am learning to be clearer about my priorities and more in touch with my own needs and preferences.

My midlife journey continues. My personal and professional growth and creativity are intertwined. Much has changed, but the words I wrote when I was 40 still express my feelings about midlife:

> The here and the now have become all important
> each moment, each gesture has its own worth.
> Life has assumed through the knowledge of dying
> a shape and a form whose only true measure is
> not length and not pleasure
> but a fullness made up of both laughter and tears.

REFERENCES

Bernard, J. *The future of marriage.* New York: Bantam, 1972.
Dinnerstein, D. *The mermaid and the minotaur: Sexual arrangements and human malaise.* New York: Harper and Row, 1977 (paperback).

Horney, K. *Feminine psychology.* New York: W. W. Norton, 1967.

Kaplan, A., & Beam, J. (Eds.). *Beyond sex-role stereotypes: Toward a psychology of androgyny.* Boston: Little Brown, 1976.

Laing, R. D. *The divided self.* London: Tavistock Publications, 1950.

Martin, D. *Battered Wives.* San Francisco: Glide, 1976.

Miller, J. B. *Toward a new psychology of women.* Boston: Beacon, 1976.

Miller, J. B. (Ed.). *Psychoanalysis and women.* Baltimore: Penguin, 1975.

Rich, A. *Of woman born.* New York: Bantam, 1977.

Rich, A. *On lies, secrets and silence.* New York: W. W. Norton, 1979.

Rich, A. Compulsory heterosexuality and lesbian experience. *Signs: Journal of women in culture and society,* 1980, *5,* 4, 631-660.

Seidenberg, R. The trauma of eventlessness. In J. B. Miller (Ed.), *Psychoanalysis and women.* Baltimore: Penguin, 1973.

Siegel, R. Women at Midlife. In *Counseling and Values,* 1982, *26,* 2, 111-117.

Walker, L. E. *The Battered Woman.* New York: Harper and Row, 1979.

Szasz, T. S. *The myth of mental illness.* New York: Dell, 1961.

Szasz, T. S. *The ethics of psychoanalysis.* New York: Dell, 1965.

Openings

Sandra Butler

This is a piece that chronicles my openings. They were many and took many forms. Some were openings outward into the world and others were inward to places deeply couched within my heart and mind. Some resulted in awareness, some in terror causing lack of speech and ability to move; but most were those of everyday stuff. I went back to my journal for clues that would help me trace my openings and found there instead the theme of silence. It has marked both my personal as well as my political and public life. The silence of well-behaved acquiescence. The silence of not knowing what sounds to shape through my lips. The silence of being afraid I was the only one. For most of my first three decades, I did not draw attention to what I came to believe was my own personal struggle and loss. Becoming a lesbian has not only given me permission to speak, but insisted that I do. Even to shout and if necessary to scream. My days of silence, punctuated only by occasional whispers has ended.

This process has been a series of small moments that happened almost without my having noticed change implicit in them. I have been a member of a political cell and have been in therapy. I have looked to my childhood as well as to the childhoods of the Third World. The answers and insights I have gained from both form the dialectic of my openings. Although the autobiographical particulars are unique to my own life, the cultural forces that shaped me also connected me to the larger pattern of women's development and sense of our shared history.

I suffered through adolescence during the early fifties, a decade where social rules insisting upon sameness shaped the lives of girl-children of the middle classes. However, by the time I was thirteen I

The author is a Bay Area writer, counselor and trainer for both professional and grass-roots organizations on issues of sexual assault and incest.

I want to particularly thank Barbara Rosenblum who helped me develop many of the ideas in this piece, and was always there to catch me if I fell.

had reached the horrifying size of six feet and one hundred forty pounds, and it was quite clear to me and my family that I was never going to be the "same" as other girls. I was called a "long drink of water," treated as an outsider and a freak, causing my family to become confused and frightened. Their solution was for me to pretend to be like everybody else while understanding that such a thing could never be possible. I read pamphlets that instructed me to wear flat shoes and never dress in stripes that go up and down. THEY DRAW ATTENTION TO YOUR HEIGHT was written in capital letters. I was further told to wear grey and navy and brown to make me appear shorter. Dates, when offered, could be accepted only by those boys taller than I. I was trapped in a body and a historical period that permitted no room for a maturation process that allowed for "small" feelings of dependency or neediness in a "big" person.

Only intermittently rebellious, I remained silent and hidden inside my flesh. My friends were characters in the books I read endlessly, my dreams filled with romantic images of handsome princes of at least six feet three waiting patiently for the opportunity to awaken me with a kiss. I was quite solitary and scarcely dared even write my feelings in my diary since to do so would be to give them a kind of acknowledgment that was too dangerous. The sounds within me that wanted to shriek of my sameness, my loneliness, my eagerness to belong and fit in, at any cost, were never uttered. I married at eighteen never really having spoken at all.

I entered the world of married adults and within the first two years eagerly produced two daughters who were to serve a variety of functions. They were to be warm and open, reflecting well on me; and by implication, on my husband as well. They were to give my life meaning and make me a successful woman. They were also to provide the only avenue to my own autonomy. My daughters were my personal act of creation and I placed the burden of creating myself upon their narrow shoulders as well.

As the decade ended, all that was required of me was that I be pliant, charming and keep most of my growing thoughts and ideas to myself. My life was carefully choreographed and the budding thinking of young brides was neither sought after nor encouraged. My daughters grew in direct proportion to the shrinking of the marriage that had produced them. My home grew around me, dwarfing me and after eight years, all fifteen rooms were filled. There was no longer space for another chair, another sofa, another vase of freshly cut flowers from the garden. The house had triumphed and it was full, glistening and richly designed. I walked among its rooms feeling as empty and unused as it was.

My husband was fifteen years older than I and I was convinced of his sophistication and worldliness in nearly all matters. Our lovemaking, however, was conducted two or three times a month. In the dark. In a hurry. And in silence. I believed that my clitoris was too "far" from my vagina and that was precisely why I had so little feeling during intercourse. I wasn't even surprised by this further proof of my physical differentness; but since it wasn't as readily visible as my size, kept it utterly to myself.

After several years of marriage, I purposefully set out to have an affair, needing to know once and for all if I was so completely unlike other women in my feelings and responses to sex. I met a man at one of the political meetings I had begun to attend. Meetings that were an outgrowth of the civil rights movement reaching even into placid suburban communities. He was dark and compelling; everything the romantic stereotypic notions that shaped my generation encouraged me to believe was sexy. He was also timely and opportunistic and we began our affair almost at once. It was acrobatic, gymnastic, lengthy, noisy and sometimes even pleasurable. But the questions remained. Why couldn't I relax? And why did I always feel so disappointed?

The ending of the affair inevitably signaled the end of my marriage as well. I had no training, experience or allowance for sex without "love" and within months found myself alone in a large city with two children and no skills. The world finally saw me as the "adult" woman I had wanted to be, but it was with approbation. I was "divorced". . .had "poor, unfortunate children with no father," and had failed myself and them. I believed all of it to be true and allowed myself to be filled with guilt and shame about the way I had lived my twenty-four years. I cradled my silence to me, denying to myself that I still needed to be cradled, and instead cradled my newly needy daughters.

I began to build my life in accordance with the shifting rules of the decade. I was able, just barely at first, to provide a living for the three of us. I attended meetings protesting the escalating war in Vietnam, supporting the growing civil rights movement and became an early organizer for the pro-busing efforts in the public schools. This work supplied me with a new sense of my ability to convince others, organize effectively, take leadership and be powerful. I found myself moving in a larger world than that of a prematurely matronly suburban wife and mother, and I began to flourish. My passion emerged in the service of political work, issues of injustice and discrimination and the possibilities for emergence of other oppressed people. I saw myself and was seen as outside all those groupings. I was a privileged white woman who could, should and did use her skills to further the movement work. What was silent and buried within me remained unvoiced.

In political circles of the early sixties, it was required that I behave like a big, Jewish, leftie chick. I could not talk about being big. Or Jewish. Or a chick. I could, however, speak of poverty, oppression, discrimination, powerlessness and the need for self-determination for everybody else except me. I was noisy and verbal about the latter and utterly silent about the former.

It was my size that was the undoing. For even if I followed all the rules as I did a decade earlier, I was still seen as threatening. Not only was I bright, articulate, insistent and demanding politically; I was a giant chick. My internal life was still and muted in order to appear safe and allow those around me to feel comfortable. I struggled to diminish myself even as I fought to grow larger in the world. And it was a silent struggle and one that took most of my energy.

With the beginnings of the movement, then called "sexual liberation," I was encouraged to be "free" of my hang-ups, my bourgeois values, and my stand-offish behaviors. This was ideally to result in me, and all women, being more available to more men, more often. It was, I was assured, the only way I could be a really politically correct comrade.

I began to experiment sexually in awkward and quite unsatisfying ways, feeling consistently that my body was out of shape and any possibility of sexual satisfaction was quite out of the question. Except, of course, for the masturbatory pleasures I had finally discovered, replete with scattered and guiltily dismissed images of large women's breasts and thighs. I tried to conform yet again, and "expressed" myself sexually as "freely" and as often as I "wanted" to. Limited, of course, to the men who would risk such a "big chick." For some, it was a challenge, but for most, a threat. I was also quite unaware of what I "wanted" and allowed by sexual encounters to be determined by my relief at being sought after and desired, however briefly. None of this halting and sporadic sexual activity was able to mask my unspoken but growing feelings of being sexually used, dismissed, diminished and trivialized. And there was no forum in which to give voice to my internal uncertainty at this measure of my "freedom" and "liberation." I had finally come to feel that my sexual "self" was unable to be satisfied. Even satin sheets, love oils, natural passions (heightened by drugs), and undemandingness with sometimes insensitive or abrupt and casual partners, were just not meant to satisfy me. I withdrew sexually to the safety, pleasure and certainty of my very tender and attentive hand. The frenzy of political and sexual activity had utterly masked the sound of my own life still caught in my throat.

On a rainy Wednesday at a meeting of the Peace and Freedom Party where Eldridge Cleaver was presenting himself as a candidate for President, my political life ended for a time. My youngest daughter had fallen asleep on the hard aluminum chair, slipping onto the lap of her sister who was awkwardly trying to complete her homework due the next morning. I was exhausted, cold, hungry. . . having rushed from work to be on time at this gathering. I leaned over, gathered up my daughters, our belongings and left.

The end of the sixties brought the beginnings of adolescence for my daughters, a partially satisfying period of solitude for me and the start of the Women's Movement. Reading was a habit born in my childhood bringing an ever-growing circle of friends who greeted me warmly into their lives and were always in readiness for my return. I returned to my beloved novels, poetry, short stories in private. To discuss them had always meant to assess their political correctness, or to detach to assess the structure of the form. I had not yet found others with whom to be joyful about skill and subtlety with language and how it shapes feelings into recognizable patterns. None with whom I could risk speaking and being "wrong" or "stupid." So I sat each night after work and read until asleep.

When the first few books presenting the early ideas of women's liberation were published, I read them with hesitancy and a sense of danger. For didn't I have the "feeling with no name"? Didn't I feel uneasy when reading about depictions of my life by male writers where I couldn't recognize myself at all? Wasn't I silent and silenced and anxious to please, even through my transformations from dutiful daughter to dutiful wife to dutiful leftie? But I was drawn to the sound of parts of my life being uttered by other women for the first time. The suspicion was born in me that I might be one of many. Not an outcast needing to be compliant and fitting in. . .not drawing attention to herself. . .not speaking bold stripes that go up and down, but speaking in grey and muted whispers.

I went to my first meeting of the "women's group" in my neighborhood just as soon as the announcement was posted on the library wall. The library that I haunted every few days for more and more books that sounded my experience. I was lonely, and anxious for a sense of belonging to a larger world than that of myself and my daughters. I hoped to find other women who would say aloud the sounds I was just barely murmuring to myself; language that made me feel less alone. A place to fit in and to belong finally. But I had no sense of what to expect. What exactly was consciousness-raising? Who were these women going to be? And I was hesitant to go because I feared the dykes there. The dyke I was to become. I dressed in fear of the neighborhood where the meeting was to be held, covering my body in an army jacket, sunglasses, cap and hiking boots. I was quite convinced that I was dressed for safety on the street in my "tough" uniform. Only later was I to discover that my appearance frightened the other women into thinking me the dyke they feared themselves.

There were nine of us at that first meeting and we met in a small room with little light and thick nervous smoke, faded cotton carpeting worn thin and covered with large pillows. As we awkwardly settled upon them, the leader said we were to go around in a circle and speak as much or as little as we wanted about why we were there and what we hoped would happen. For me, this was the first time I began with the truth. . .intimacy, something I had always parceled out carefully and only after much testing. While I was prepared to "tell the truth," I had developed elaborate skills in presenting the "truth" in a charming, entertaining and anecdotal way so that these new women would like me and perhaps become my friends. I scarcely heard those who spoke before me, I was so busy in sorting and shifting through my images so that they were polished and smooth.

They spoke haltingly, as unused as I to being listened to, and truly heard. It began to occur to me that no one was going to be interrupted, or challenged, questioned or evaluated, I began straining to understand what it was that was going on. While I grew frightened and confused, there was an excitement that began in my chest until, when it was my turn to speak, I cried in relief in front of these women. . .something entirely new for me. Women I had never known before, never tested for safety, never assessed as to their political correctness. Their words called up the shared images of women whose lives reflected bitterness and denial. Many of the faces conjured up for me were the closed, set, pinched ones of women who never lived, except within the grimly circumscribed lives they were permitted. Each face I saw in my mind's eye was singular, but the eyes sometimes blurred. They became eyes that held a banked fury masked by the language women have learned to speak. It is a language of accommodation, of yielding, of self-mutilation. It was the language of much my own life as well. I had diminished my body, my options, my expressiveness and had spent my life being well-behaved. And never pleasing anyone. Myself least of all.

That meeting was for me the beginning of congruence, the beginning of speech and the beginning of community. The early awkwardnesses began to fade after several meetings and the trust never before experienced with other women began to form. I began to hear echoes of my own well-behaved compliance attached to the hopes of being acceptable. . .belonging. I learned that other men admonished women not to be so "emotional." I understood that who I was had been shaped by my family and body, as well as by a deeply mysogynistic culture. I began to know that my body was not unusual and that the precise distance from clitoris to vaginal opening was not my unique shame. And that sexual pleasure was not automatic and experienced by everybody else except me. We spoke together in a language that was softer and more expressive than any I had heard before, or read before or imagined before. And it provided a safety for me to utter my secrets and not fear the horror that greets outcasts and misfits. The unsaid and unlit corners of my experience became illuminated.

It was the beginning of a new way to think about healing and nurturing. It was the creation of a new form and it was the genesis of my becoming whole. We struck the most delicate balance between demanding and insisting on the fullest and finest from each of us, and carefully and painstakingly helping each other move through our terrors and feelings of inadequacy. We were re-thinking what it meant to be fully alive. Fully human. A woman. And I was never the same again.

But it was not only feeling together that moved me forward into speech. For we also were thinking together. Reformulating the world in a language and theory that reflected our experiences as women. We were shaping an understanding of gender relations. My years of reading and writing and thinking gave me courage to speak and I found another part of my voice. That of an analytic and thoughtful woman who could think emotionally, and cerebrally as well, and see connections to her personal and cultural rages.

Within a year I had begun college (at thirty-five), bringing to it the strength, sense of increased certainty, skills and all the delayed passion of the late-bloomer. The decade of the 70s was one of possibilities for women, and for me as well, a deepening and opening of all my possibilities that had remained buried under my "well-behaved" silence.

My interest and commitment to writing intensified and I used language to explain my own trajectory into the welcoming arms of "our" movement. I wrote to understand what I thought and I wrote to share what I felt in the constantly shifting relationship between the internal and external world of my own experience. My life was nearly populated solely by women. I used my organizing skills to begin a teaching collective and learned how the process of women doing work together was every bit as important as the work itself; quite different from the goal orientation of the political groups of the sixties. I understood how the ways in which we are together as women inform the nature and the quality of the work we do and the personal success we can feel doing it.

I brought all these growing insights and budding strengths into my few relationships with men and found the magnitude of the importance of these changes in me, and their liberating qualities made no impact on the men other than to intensify their anger and insecurity. Now I had become the castrating bitch of their worst dreams. Here before them was a man-hating, ball-busting, demanding, insistent, "women's libber." Only now, I knew it wasn't me that was wrong. I could now understand the sources of their terror and rage; place it in both its personal as well as political context, and withdraw whole and intact from the encounter.

There were exceptions, of course. Men who were warm and loving and anxious to "understand" and be "supportive." And I am grateful for them, for they helped me to know that they were the exceptions and the outcasts. Not me.

I immersed myself totally in the community of women and my heart and flesh responded. To all the women at first and finally to one woman in particular. And then another. And then a growing sense that this was a natural outgrowth of my path. I remember so clearly thinking how "natural" it all finally was. The congruence of work, thought, action, feeling, laughter and flesh. With women.

I am learning and re-learning how to be a big woman, a woman who insists and demands, and is often not well-behaved, as well as a woman who allows herself to be small, protected and nurtured. A Jew who struggles with the confusing and uneasy alliances of

Zionism and the vision of a world without borders. A woman who tries to juggle time for writing and time for political activity. A mother with a mother who is aging, 3,000 miles away and alone. A white woman whose class privilege allowed the development of skills that supported me and my children during their early years. A lesbian who takes joy in the robust strength of women; their subtlety and grace; their flesh and their passion and their insistence on radical transformation. No one identity subsumes or diminishes the importance of the other. And each has time to be central.

I am not a "country dyke," wearing flannel clothes and constructing a primary relationship with the land; I am not a devotee of "women's music," I go to fewer and fewer rallies and demonstrations. I do not have a category within which to define myself as a lesbian. And I don't want one. I have shared with thousands of women a background of choices made in failed marriages, primary care for children, political work, emotional isolation and uncertainty, rage at the "isms" that diminish human possibility. And I insist that my life and its choices move me closer to, rather than away from, our shared humanity. I will no longer be smaller than I am, nor permit my life to be diminished by others in the name of their own ideology.

It is too late for me to be a particular kind of lesbian, for the compromise, accommodation, denial and yielding have already cost me parts of myself that are nearly irretrievable. I am a lesbian. It is a way to live that reflects my love of and for women; a way to structure my time, interests and concerns with those of other women; a way to fill myself with the energy and sweetness of women.

Each dimension of my life is grounded in loving women. Loving myself as a woman. And I will continue to write and speak and insist and struggle. A lesbian is a woman who loves woman. And I most surely do.

Hispanic Women:
Stress and Mental Health Issues

Guadalupe Gibson

INTRODUCTION

To speak of Hispanic women in the United States is to refer to:

> . . .an amalgam of millions of persons from a variety of races,
> religions, and political and cultural experiences (who) are
> through historical circumstances or political or individual
> design, a permanent and vital segment of our population (and)
> who are striving to improve their status in this society, while
> maintaining their dignity and identity in both cultures (Con-
> ference on the Educational and Occupational Needs of His-
> panic Women, 1980, p. 7).

Hispanic is a generic label for a diverse group of Spanish-
speaking and/or Spanish-surnamed people in the United States, who
reflect various histories, ethnic backgrounds and, therefore, a wide
range of values. There is not only considerable inter-group diversity, but there is also marked and significant intra-group heterogeneity (LeVine & Padilla, 1980). Included among the Hispanics are
Puerto Ricans, Cubans, and Mexican Americans, the groups most
easily identifiable; as well as Central and South Americans, Domin-
icans, and others. Chicanos who constitute the largest sub-group,
are primarily concentrated in the Southwest, the Puerto Ricans
mostly in the Northeast, and the Cubans in the Southeast. Hispanics
are now considered to be the second-largest minority group in the

The author is Professor at the Worden School of Social Service, Our Lady of the Lake
University, and Director, La Chicana & Mental·Health, NIMH Project, 1976-1981.

113

United States, but they may constitute the largest minority group by the turn of the century ("It's your turn in the sun," 1978).

Most Hispanic women in spite of the heterogeneity among them, share similar concerns about maintaining their language and cultural identity and a commonality of experiences as a "minority" group within the dominant society, primarily their involvement is in the persistent confrontation with the manifestations of racism, the most pernicious of which is generalized poverty (LeVine & Padilla, 1980; Melville, 1980a). Hispanic women also share, as all American women do, their struggles with the issues of equity and their victimization due to sexism.

This paper will identify the multiple sources of psychological stress that impinge on Hispanic women, will address the mental health problems that they generally experience, and will describe interventive approaches and preventive strategies that take their linguistic and cultural needs, as well as their socioeconomic circumstances into consideration. Some emphasis will be given to the problems of Mexican American women, the group with whom I am intimately familiar.

BACKGROUND

It is essential to understand the historical background and other facts about various Hispanic groups in order to understand their status as minority people. Because most Hispanics are *mestizos,* a product of racial mixtures, Caucasian—Spanish, Portuguese, and others—with indigenous groups and Blacks, they have been considered a "population of color," and have been subjected to racist discrimination (Jimenez-Vazquez, 1980; LeVine & Padilla, 1980).

Even a cursory review of the literature reveals that Anglo researchers and social scientists, using an ethnocentric, assimilative perspective, based on the mythological philosophy of the "melting pot," have portrayed Hispanics derogatorily, and described Hispanic families stereotypically. Their behaviors and family life-styles have been considered deviant and/or pathological, caused by their tenacious adherence to their language and culture. These generalizations have been made from small samples which included mainly people from rural areas and poor urban barrios, which reflected the problems of people who were impoverished and who had not had access to adequate resources or services (Gibson, 1978; Montiel, 1970; Romano, I., 1973; Romano, O., 1973; Vaca, 1970). These same so-called "authorities," also proposed policy that was damaging to Hispanics because it ran counter to the behaviors valued by them. For example,

> . . . public policy discouraged bilingualism, encouraged segregation, ignored inequality and maintained welfare rules that disrupted family life. The perspective underlying such policy was detached, corrective, and invariably punitive (Montiel, 1978, p. xi).

Since the civil rights movements, the situation has improved considerably. There are now more Hispanic researchers and social scientists who are more accurately perceiving Hispanic families, but some victims of such policies and their children are still suffering the consequences.

The portrayal of Hispanic women in social science literature has been even worse than that of Hispanics in general. There has been even less valid field research, theoretical work, or compiled information on them. Information that is available is mostly inaccurate and appears to be biased (Andrade, 1981b & c; Conference. . . , 1980; Melville, 1980a; Mirande & Enriquez, 1979; Senour, 1977). They are depicted as mother figures, self-sacrificing, passive, pleased and obliged to produce large families, living within rigidly defined sex roles, and dominated by the males. These portrayals of Hispanic women are being challenged by more recent studies conducted primarily by Hispanics, some of them women. Cromwell and Ruiz (1979) undertook an intensive analysis of four major studies on decision-making in Mexican and Mexican American families to examine the male dominance concept. They concluded that the available empirical evidence did not substantiate the hypothesis of male dominance in marital decision-making. The data they reviewed suggested that:

> Hispanic males may behave differently from non-Hispanic males in their family and marital lives, but of course, not in the inappropriate fashion suggested by the myth with its strong connotation of social deviance (p. 371).

Andrade (1981c) identified other major studies on marital decision-making which also failed to support the hypothesis of *machismo* or male dominance. These studies of family dynamics revealed that when couples were interviewed in regard to decision-making, action-taking, marital satisfaction, the employment of wives, and egalitarianism, the assumed dominance of the men and submissiveness of the women did not hold at all. Other persisting stereotypes are also being dispelled, such as those in regard to attitudes and behaviors about family planning and abortion (Amaro, 1980; Andrade, 1980, 1981a; Garcia, 1980; Garcia-Bahne, 1977; Salazar, 1979, 1980; Urdaneta, 1980). The picture that seems to be emerging is that of a population of women who are attempting, with varying degrees of success, to move into the mainstream of American life without losing their cultural identity.

In spite of their concern about sexist oppression and other feminist issues, Hispanic women have found it difficult to identify with the Women's Movement. They have tended to be suspicious of it because they believe that issues of race and class have been obscured by sexual politics, and they have seen little evidence of white women attempting to understand, much less address, the broader needs of minority women (Hart, 1977; Nieto, 1974). They have gradually formulated their own feminist ideology which shares some of the goals of the white feminists, but which has some distinct characteristics. Chicanas see feminism as structurally and ideologically integrated with the Chicano Movement for the enhancement of power and status of all Hispanics. It reaffirms intra-group solidarity and places a strong emphasis on the family. Because it calls for the participation of entire families in political action, Zinn (1975b) refers to it as political familism which facilitates sex role equality in the family (Cotera, 1973, 1980; Mason, 1980; Mirande & Enriquez, 1979; Zinn, 1975a). It is compatible with what appear to be conflicting goals "of the preservation of traditional culture and the eradication of traditional patterns of female subordination" (Mason, 1980, p. 106). New conceptualizations of the female and male ideals are being formulated: a woman who respects men, the family and the home, but is able to combine this with opportunities for higher education, work outside the home, and with social and political activities in the community, and a man who identifies with the positive aspects of *machismo,* is flexible, respects women and his family, and can share in the successes of women (Mason, 1980; Rendon, 1971). Chicanos and other Hispanic men are reflecting this ideology as well (Mason, 1975; Terrones, 1977; Zinn, 1975a).

Current literature reflects that the roles of Hispanic women are changing. The number of those in the labor force has increased;

more have attained higher education; some have earned doctoral degrees. They are employed in such diverse fields as construction, education, management, engineering, law and medicine. A few hold elected political offices, are employed at various levels of government, or have been appointed to significant governmental positions such as Marilucy Jaramillo, who recently served as U. S. Ambassador to Honduras. Many are married and are enjoying the full support of their husbands. Hispanic families range from the very poor to the very rich, including a few millionaires, but they continue to be disproportionately poor; 25 percent of them are reported below the poverty level. One in six Hispanic families is headed by a woman, and one out of every two of these exists below the poverty level. In spite of changes Hispanic women continue to lack academic credentials and work skills because of limited educational and vocational opportunities (Hart, 1977; Vivo, 1981).

Hispanics are characterized by diversity among and within the various subgroups, but they share common socio-cultural elements which bind them as Hispanics, principally the cultural heritage of Spain and the Spanish language. They share a number of values, cultural attributes, and demographic characteristics. Their most important commonality is the significance of the family which has been pivotal for them. The concept of family is not limited to the nuclear family, but goes beyond to the extended family and embraces *compadres,* neighbors, and friends. These kinship ties have enabled them to survive in what has often been a hostile environment (Alvirez & Bean, 1976; Fitzpatric, 1976; Garcia-Bahne, 1977; Gilbert, 1978; Gutierrez, 1979; Murillo, 1972).

Hispanics continue to be predominantly Catholic, although many have not been active in the Church. Until the recent "latinization" of the Church, many saw it as ethnocentric, oppressive, and even as a racist institution. As the number of Hispanic priests grows and services are provided in Spanish, more people have become active in the church again. The number of Hispanic Protestants is growing as Protestant churches have accelerated their evangelization efforts among them, are recruiting Hispanics to provide charismatic ministry, and are offering services in Spanish. Regardless of denomination or unorthodoxy, religion continues to be a central element within their culture, and as a whole, they are highly spiritual. Many social activities center around religion (Benitez, 1980; Dieppa & Montiel, 1978; Lara-Braud, 1971; LeVine & Padilla, 1980; Martinez, 1978; Sandoval, 1978).

LANGUAGE AND CULTURE

Most Hispanics have maintained Spanish as their primary language. First generation Hispanics usually speak little or no English, and since the extended family ties remain strong, the use of the language is reinforced. Some Hispanics are monolingual in Spanish; others are monolingual in English. The majority of them are bilingual to a greater or lesser degree; that is, they use both languages with varying degrees of understanding and proficiency, and they do not always have parallel vocabularies. Some Hispanics speak a patois or dialectal Spanish (Gomez & Cerda, 1976).

Culturally, some Hispanics have retained their Hispanic culture almost intact; others have been assimilated, but on occasion display vestiges of their Hispanic culture. The majority are bicultural, having synthesized—in some instances syncretized—the Hispanic and the Anglo American cultures. While attempting to retain the core of their culture, they have been flexible and adaptable and have developed values that are functional within their environment (Dieppa & Montiel, 1978; Gomez & Cerda, 1976). Some have been able to modify the behavioral expressions of some values in accommodating to new situations and have discarded other values which are no longer functional (Fallis, 1976).

The bicultural experience signifies participation, though differently, in the two cultural systems and within two sets of behaviors. This characterization of *dual response* which according to Chestang (1972) has both conscious and unconscious aspects, and which is internalized as a central aspect of the personality, does not mean dual personality; rather it involves two distinct ways of coping with tasks, expectations and behaviors. The dual responses converge within the person as an integrated whole (Ibid). For example, an Hispanic woman may behave cooperatively at home with her family and friends as her culture demands, but she can behave competitively in the employment setting as the Anglo American culture requires. Biculturalism gives people alternative modes for behaviors under different circumstances (Ulibarri, undated).

SOURCES OF STRESS
AND MENTAL HEALTH PROBLEMS

Stress is a normal, inevitable part of life. The only complete freedom from stress is death. It is experienced in family relations, moving about in traffic, shopping, and dealing with countless human problems and situations, including happy events—getting married, graduating, even getting a raise. How much of a burden all of these stressors become depends on the frequency, the duration and the intensity of the various stressors; the demands that each places on the individual; and on the number of stressors the person has to cope with simultaneously (Bauman, 1980; Freese, 1980). Even though some experts believe that there is both good and bad stress, that some level of stress may be beneficial and even essential to mobilize people to take positive action, to be productive, and to achieve goals, most experts agree that there is no such thing as good stress. Regardless of what kind, if stress is constant and prolonged, it can be devastating to the person's physical and emotional health (Bauman, 1980; Freese, 1980). The psychosocial effects of society on the mind and emotions of individuals was recognized by Wolff as early as 1953 (Fried, 1982). Ongoing studies and new research are reinforcing the conclusions he drew, that certain groups of people are at risk because of stress, among whom are members of low-status ethnic minorities, women, the elderly and the poor (Bauman, 1980). In addition to being victims of chronic persistent stress or distress, these individuals are incapable of modifying their relationship to the sources of their stressful conditions, or to their environment, and have few options, if any, to deal with stress. Even those who have the capacity to meet the challenge, to identify and use other resources, often do not have a single resource available to them. They may find such circumstances difficult to accept, but are powerless to change them. The sense of powerlessness is the most significant source of stress and the most difficult to combat (Ibid.).

HISPANIC WOMEN AND STRESS

Without doubt Hispanic women suffer psychological stress because of sexism as all other American women do. As minority women, they suffer additional stress because of adverse social conditions, overt and covert prejudice, pervasive poverty, extremely high unemployment and/or underemployment, overcrowded and delapidated housing, poor health, difficulty with English fluency, stresses inherent in acculturation, and numerous other environmental stresses (Boulette, 1976a; Hasell, 1980; LeVine & Padilla, 1980). Some of these stressors affect all Hispanic women regardless of sub-group identity or socioeconomic status. Others most significantly impact the poor.

One general problem for Hispanic women is related to their poor self-concept and low self-esteem. They have been conditioned through the educational process and other negative experiences, both as women and as members of a minority group, to believe that they are inept, incapable, and that they should limit their aspirations (Melville, 1980a). Ambassador Jaramillo (1980) has recounted her experiences which raised self-doubts and made her question her ability. She urged Hispanic women to fight their feelings of insecurity and avoid setting themselves up to fail. Although there appears to be some improvement in this area as more appropriate role models emerge, Hispanic women continue to be plagued by self-doubts.

Acculturation is a complex process which occurs when a group of people having a different culture from that of a host society, change or modify some of their original cultural patterns and absorb some of the prevailing cultural patterns of the majority culture in order to accommodate to the new environment. This process can be prolonged and quite painful (Arce & Torres-Matrullo, 1980). For Hispanic women acculturation can be a multifaceted, intergenerational problem, regardless of their socioeconomic status. It can be particularly severe for those older women who are recent arrivals or who have had limited educational experiences in the United States. Many find themselves in conflict with their children (Canino & Canino, 1980; LeVine & Padilla, 1980; Szapocznic & Truss, 1978). Marked conflict often occurs between mothers and their young adult daughters who want to attend universities or seek better job opportunities away from home; who want to work or go back to school even though married and with children; who choose not to marry but elect to live with a man. Alienation from the family is very stressful for younger Hispanic women, for even though they have a different perception of the family, family ties are still important to them. In an open letter to her mother a young Puerto Rican let her know how some of her values had changed and how others were in the process of changing, and by so doing confirmed her need for the relationship with her. She stated:

> I want to introduce you to these new values we do not share, and in so doing, we will begin communicating woman to woman, not exclusively mother to daughter. Hiding this new dimension of me is an awkward feeling, and I must rely on being real with myself and with you (Marrero, 1978, p. 69).

She then described what her new values were. So many women are not able to face conflicts with their parents as this woman does. They acquiesce and give up their strivings, or sever their relationships, often suffering emotionally and even physically.

An even more serious acculturation problem that some Hispanic women have to face is that of conflict with their spouses. The most prevalent one seems to be that between a wife who has acculturated and who may even consider herself liberated, and her husband who retains, if not all his traditional values, at least some pertaining to marital and family relationships. At times, she may have to be an advocate for the children who may want more freedom than a traditional father is willing to give. If a woman chooses to work, or if she has to work to make ends meet, her husband may make it very clear that he will "allow" her to do so as long as she keeps up with her "obligations" as wife and mother. She not only has to cope with stress on the job, but with that at home as well. Quarrels may be easily triggered, even violence may result. Her options are limited to whether she stays in the marriage or chooses to divorce. If she divorces, she then faces perhaps an even more stressful situation as a single mother head of the household. This alternative could even cause her to become alienated from her family who may agree with her husband's point of view. There are many variations of acculturation problems between husbands and wives, most of them especially stressful to the wife.

The stresses created by migrancy need to be recognized. Puerto Ricans, who ordinarily move to the mainland for economic reasons, do suffer cultural shock when they arrive. They have to compete with United States residents for dwindling low-paying jobs, often lack English fluency, have difficulty finding adequate housing, and generally the whole experience is tremendously stressful for the family. The women bear the burden of keeping the family stable. They often succeed in getting a job before their husbands do, and they support the men through the indignities of being deprived of a job, helping them to maintain their self-esteem. They encourage the children to attend and remain in school and carry the major responsibility for their care and for all the household chores. Some succeed, others suffer emotionally and/or physically. The stresses for other immigrant women are just as severe, often more so than those experienced by resident Hispanics.

Those who enter the United States illegally, euphemistically referred to as the undocumented, usually settle in large urban centers or join the migrant stream. Because they have to avoid discovery and, therefore, deportation, their daily life becomes unbelievably distressful.

Stressful, too, is the life of the women in the migrant stream. Mexican Americans, some Puerto Ricans, a few Cubans, and other Hispanics travel yearly following the crops, usually moving northward from the southern states. Migrants are underpaid, exposed to fertilizers and other chemicals, lack adequate and sanitary housing facilities, no health services are available to them, and no appropriate schooling for their children. The women often carry major responsibility for the family care in addition to working alongside the men in the fields. They bear all the problems stoically, often portraying the stereotype—the abnegated, self-denying, self-sacrificing woman (Melville, 1980b; Solis, 1972).

Job related stress for all Hispanic women in the work-force is similar to that experienced by all American women—last hired, first fired, tokenism, less pay for equal work, sexual harassment, and all other known stressors due to sexism. But they also experience greater discrimination as minority women. The rate of unemployment and underemployment is much higher for them, and they earn even less money that white women do. The median income for Mexican American women in 1976 was roughly three fourths of that for all women. One out of three Chicanas and one out of five Puerto Ricans, many of whom are raising their children alone, earned less than $2,000 a year (Anguiano, 1979; Melville, 1980a). Other discriminatory practices in employment that affect Hispanic women are related to the stereotypic view of them as lazy, undependable and inadequate (Melville, 1980a). Another factor that affects their employment is that of language. Some do not speak English; others lack fluency, and still others, though fluent, speak with an accent. This may deprive them of certain job opportunities, regardless of how well prepared they are for the jobs they seek. They may not be told why, but they do not get the job. There are some women's training programs that categorize Hispanic women who have an accent and a dark complexion as handicapped.

Poor Hispanic women who have usually lacked economic stability over the years and probably come from a family of origin that was also poor, share long-range socio-psychological and health problems related to prolonged economic deprivation. The pressures most of these women have to bear seem almost insurmountable. Many of them have not finished school, married early, and have a number of children. They usually have no skills, and if employed, have to work in the most menial jobs with no future. Those who are on welfare have a meager income, for most states do not provide grants that cover even the minimum necessary to meet basic human needs. If they enroll in work-training programs, child care facilities are often inadequate, and they may have no family support systems. Their relatives may not live nearby or may be living in similar circumstances and are unable to help. These are the women that may resort to drink and drug abuse, or to violence through child abuse, and for whom mental health services may not be available.

MENTAL HEALTH SERVICES
FOR HISPANIC WOMEN

Hispanic women, particularly those who are poor, undoubtedly experience a great deal of endemic stress, a condition caused by continuous and manifold changes, demands, threats, or deprivations frequently small in scale and embedded in daily life events (Lazarus, 1981). They must, therefore, be in need of mental health services. Yet, until fairly recently, Hispanics have generally underutilized mental health services (Burruel & Chavez, 1974; Chavez, 1979; Phillipus, 1971). Padilla (1975) and others, have emphasized that the policies of mental health facilities have been discouraging to Hispanics; that there are language barriers and cultural and class disparity between the clients and the therapists; and most importantly, that the standard approach to the provision of services has been anchored in white, middle-class value-based theoretical frames of reference. The focus has been on intrapsychic problems, with emphasis on changing the individual while ignoring the environment which often triggered the maladaptive behaviors (Burruel & Chavez, 1974; Fischer, 1978; Gibson, 1977; Keefe, 1978; Morales, 1978; Padilla & Ruiz, 1973; Ruiz et al., 1977; Torrey, 1970).

During the past ten or twelve years considerable improvement has been made as practitioners have been moving away from ethnocentric treatment approaches, but particularly since the number of Hispanic mental health service providers has increased. There are now a number of Hispanic research centers conducting meaningful research on the mental health needs of Hispanics. The Spanish Speaking Mental Health Research Center, Los Angeles, which publishes the *Hispanic Journal of Behavioral Sciences,* and the Hispanic

Research Center at Fordham University, New York, are but two examples. The number of scholarly works, including dissertations, continues to grow, contributing to the further understanding of Hispanics and their circumstances in the United States. New therapeutic models, particularly for family therapy, are being created, adaptations of traditional theoretical frameworks are being discovered, and the results of these approaches are being analyzed (LeVine & Padilla, 1980; Padilla & Ruiz, 1973). However, literature on specific interventions for Hispanic women is still meager. Boulette (1976 a & b) has discussed assertiveness training, therapeutic listening and behavioral rehearsal with low income Mexican American women; Hynes and Werbin (1977) have described group psychotherapy with Spanish-speaking women; and Szapocznic and Truss (1978) analyzed their work with Cuban mothers experiencing role conflict. Services to Hispanic women are mostly provided through family therapy, which in most instances is appropriate.

In my own practice, both in a mental health clinic and in private practice, I found that an eclectic approach was the most effective. I often had to use a variety of interventive strategies in order to address all the problems that some of the Mexican American women presented. It is often necessary to advocate and to intercede for them to bring about change. I worked with some women on welfare whose children were not receiving free lunches because the family had "regular income." After a series of meetings with the School Board and the administrators, changes were made that included the "Welfare Families" in the school lunch programs.

I found role playing a very effective approach to treatment with some women to demonstrate what they could do, or for me to get a better picture of what was happening in the family. A case of a middle-aged woman who brought her son to the clinic because he was acting out in school is an example. The father, a truck driver, could not come in as he was often out of town, and when in town he refused to come in. All the sessions were conducted bilingually as she could express herself better by using both languages interchangeably. She had only a fifth grade education and no education in Spanish. She depicted her husband as a weekend heavy drinker, bossy and unconcerned about their five children. She described his behavior when he came in from trips as hostile, demanding and not interested in how the family had fared while he was gone. We role-played both her behavior and his. When I role-played the husband as she had described him, she could admit that perhaps she exaggerated how he comported himself. When I played her role, I demonstrated both how she acted helpless and nagged consistently, and how she could be assertive. The only feed-back I was getting was what the son reported to his therapist, that his mother had gotten "off my back," and that the parents were arguing less. Approximately three months later, her husband came with her to the session saying that he wanted to meet "the woman who had set my wife's head straight." He started to come on a fairly regular basis, participated in role playing and after a few sessions stated, "My head needed to be set straight, too. I am glad I came." Both of them, as well as their son, were doing much better in a number of ways when we closed the case.

I also worked with groups of young women who were struggling to become more independent of their families. An example is a group of five women in their twenties who felt incapacitating guilt. Two were working and three others were enrolled in higher education. These women were unable to deal with their parents directly, particularly their mother, about living away from home, not coming to visit every weekend, not having to call "at least every other day" to tell their mother how they were doing. In the group they were able, with my help, to assist each other, to learn to become assertive and to accept that their families were not going to change. It was interesting that they could transfer the new behaviors to the other relationships in their lives. The two that were working were able to deal with their employers about promotions.

Another significant aspect of the group was that they could speak in English throughout most of the sessions except when they talked about their recollection of their families as they were growing up, especially about the advice—*los consejos*—that their mother gave them, particularly in terms of future heterosexual relationships. One of them said that often when she became intimate with her boyfriend she could hear her mother clearly admonishing her. These women developed considerable insight and were able to deal with the unconscious content that did surface. Fairly recent feedback from some of them has been that they are doing well intra as well as interpersonally.

The type of ethnotherapy that is being practiced by the Institute on Pluralism and Group Identity in New York with Jewish people who are struggling with identity problems would be most effective in work with Hispanic women who have become assimilated, but are distressed because of their alienation from their families.

Cultural assessment approaches and assertiveness training can be effective with women of all socioeconomic levels as Boulette (1976a and b) has demonstrated. Educational approaches from a preventive perspective can be initiated as early as at the high school level and can be implemented with elderly women. I was consultant to a program of elderly Mexican American women, most of whom were single. They were able to integrate the new knowledge and understanding into their everyday lives, particularly in dealing with their children who were overprotective of them.

IMPLICATIONS FOR PRACTICE

Attempting to provide mental health services to Hispanic women presents a real challenge to those in the mental health field. Hispanic women need services that are not discriminatory either because of their minority status or because of their gender, and which recognize and respect the heterogeneity among them—ethnic, racial, socioeconomic, level of acculturation or biculturalism, and linguistic variance. Bilingual services should be made available to Hispanic women since communication is crucial to service delivery. Problems of miscommunication may occur even when a client appears to be fluent in English. This is worse than non-communication because neither the client nor the therapist may know that they have not communicated, and may not realize that wrong information has been given and/or received. Often clients do not have parallel vocabularies or may not know various meanings of words. A person who calls saying that she is not able to keep her appointment because she broke her doll and is going to the hospital may not necessarily be having a psychotic break. She may have broken her wrist, which in Spanish is called *muñeca,* and *muñeca* also means doll, a more popular use of the term. She may have never heard of the word wrist if, for instance, she dropped out of a segregated school after the third grade.

Another important factor about language is that a person's first language is the one that ordinarily has affective meaning. They may have to use Spanish to describe intimate, gut-level issues. When speaking in English, they may appear to have flat affect, when in reality, the problem is linguistic. Often when they switch to Spanish, they become animated and display a whole range of emotions. Other linguistic problems include the fact that some concepts may be positive in one language and negative in another and neither the client nor the therapist may be aware of it (Anders et al., 1977; Kline et al., 1977). The use of interpreters may be limiting, for much of the state of the art in mental health is "gaining information from the way clients phrase their statements and questions" (Baker, 1981, p. 393). Professional interpreters may be used effectively if trained in mental health. The use of children to interpret, particularly minor ones, is inappropriate, and so is the use of neighbors and friends, and even clerical workers, unless there is an emergency. Not only is it unethical, but they may not have parallel vocabularies either, and they may misinform the client, the therapist, or both.

The subject of bilingualism is complicated and needs special attention. Therapists need to understand the phenomenon in depth. Bilingual therapists, including Hispanics themselves, must do so, too, for there are many variations of the language, from ethnic group to ethnic group, inter-generational and even regional, which may preclude adequate communication.

Understanding various components of the culture is also significant. Body language, patterns of communication and the affective meaning of certain concepts, anger, aspiration and grief, for instance, can be understood only through adequate comprehension of the culture (Vassiliou & Vassiliou, 1974). The level of acculturation of Hispanics needs to be known for a better grasp of their total reality. There are now some acculturation scales which therapists can learn to use with good results. One is intended to identify the different levels of acculturation of marital partners (Gomez, 1979; Moore, undated).

It is essential that mental health providers avoid stereotyping Hispanic women. Some of the literature is replete with stereotypes on *machismo, hembrismo,* * *marianismo,* ** and other mythic cultural expectations, which interfere with the appropriate provision of service. Nonetheless, as is true of all stereotypes, some individuals do fit them. Some Hispanic women, for instance, even some who appear to be liberated, sophisticated and modernistic, have been strongly socialized into certain traditions that enmesh them in

---

Hembrismo is a term coined by Bermudez (1955) to describe the traditional female role, the counterpart of *machismo*. *Hembra* means female.

**Maria* means Mary and *marianismo* refers to an attitude reflecting saintly attitudes such as those the Virgin Mary represents. *Marianismo* is used to describe the attitudes of self-sacrificing, self-denying women.

cultural conflicts and value dilemmas. One example of a controversial value which still appears to persist, according to Medina and Reyes (1976), is that women are expected to be "pure" and virginal when they first marry. These women need sensitive help in making the most viable decisions for themselves as to whether to retain or discard such traditions. They may need help in identifying more appropriate behavioral expressions of their values.

According to Cruz (1977), many of these women, and some Hispanic men as well, despite the popular notion of the sex role identity inherent in the *machismo/hembrismo* conceptualization, and the masculinity/femininity dichotomy in the Anglo American culture, are beginning to consider the alternative of androgyny as postulated by Bem (1975a & b). Cruz further states that androgyny, similarly to biculturalism, "emphasizes flexible diversity rather than rigid stereotypes and dichotomies" (1977, p. 2).

Another stereotype among many others is that of women who present an unusually high degree of often vague somatic complaints of physical discomfort and pain. They insist on the legitimacy of their headaches, dizziness, muscular aches, chest pains and palpitations, and explain that they would get well if they could control their "nerves" (Abad et al., 1977). Most of these women have, at best, been assumed to be denying emotional problems and were advised to seek insight psychotherapy. At worst these individuals were labeled dependent and often accused of being malingerers, attempting to get on, or to stay on welfare. New knowledge of the physical effects of stress, as stated above, substantiates their complaints as legitimate.

It is urgent that mental health practitioners identify the many strengths of Hispanic women and use these maximally in treatment. The assimilative perspective which encouraged them to discard their identification with their culture needs to be changed to one that recognizes bilingualism and biculturalism as a positive force (Ramirez, 1977). New research points to the advantages of bilingualism which enables people to develop bicognitive style, and biculturalism which provides a basis for a more flexible and sophisticated psychological adjustment (Ibid.).

Ramirez (1979) urged mental health practitioners to stop viewing *machismo* negatively as a cultural shortcoming or as male chauvinism, which is not indigenous to Hispanics. *Machismo* in its positive cultural characteristics reflects honesty, loyalty, fairness, and responsibility. He stated:

A *macho* is affectionate, hard working, amiable and family oriented. He can admit his mistakes and knows when to ask for help. By emphasizing these positive cultural characteristics, the *machismo* concept becomes a bridge, rather than a barrier, in engaging Chicanos in family or marital counseling (p. 62).

There is no better way to help Hispanic women with their mental health problems than through involvement of the men in their lives in the therapeutic process. Hispanic women tend to be optimistic, particularly because of their strong religious beliefs which provide roots of hope. This optimism is a strength that should be used in the therapeutic process.

Preventive efforts in the interest of Hispanic women need to be made as well. The most significant approach is through education. Family life education and child rearing management skills are all areas in which they are interested. They have been found to be responsive when such programs are offered to them at a time convenient to them, and in a language they can understand. The media in general can be used to disseminate the information they need. Periodicals, public affairs bulletins, and other printed materials can be used as well (Chavez, 1979).

In conclusion, it is important to say that mental health practitioners, regardless of their therapeutic orientation, should continue to explore approaches for serving Hispanic women in ways that are culturally congruent and that address their needs as women. Ultimately, as Carrillo (1978) stated, these approaches must not only help individuals deal with specific problems, but must also be capable of effecting changes in society which will enable them to be free of stress and in charge of their own destinies.

REFERENCES

Abad, V., Ramos, J., and Boyce E. Clinical issues in the psychiatric treatment of Puerto Ricans. In E. R. Padilla and A. M. Padilla (Eds.), *Transcultural Psychiatry: An Hispanic Perspective.* University of California at Los Angeles: Spanish Speaking Mental Health Research Center. 1977, 25-34.

Alvirez, D., and Bean, F. D. The Mexican-American family. In C. H. Mindel and R. W. Habenstein (Eds.), *Ethnic Families in America: Patterns Variations.* New York: Elsevier, 1976, 271-292.

Amaro, H. Abortion use and attitudes among Chicanas: The need for research. *Research Bulletin.* UCLA, Spanish Speaking Mental Health Research Center, *4,* No. 3, March 1980, 1-4.

Anders, A., Chatel, J., Parlade, R., and Pelle, R. Why we did not establish a separate complete program for Spanish speaking patients. In E. R. Padilla and A. M. Padilla (Eds.), *Transcultural Psychiatry: An Hispanic Perspective.* Monograph number four. UCLA, Spanish Speaking Mental Health Research Center. 1977, 63-66.

Andrade, S. J. Family planning practices of Mexican Americans. In M. B. Melville (Ed.), *Twice a Minority: Mexican American Women.* St. Louis: The C. V. Mosby Company, 1980, 17-32.

Andrade, S. J. Contraceptive use by adolescents: What we know about Chicanas. Paper presented in the symposium "Passages a la Mexicana," at the annual meeting of the American Education Research Association, Los Angeles, April 1981a (Mimeographed).

Andrade, S. J. Social science stereotypes of the Mexican American woman: Policy implications for research. *Hispanic Journal of Behavioral Sciences.* UCLA, Fall 1981b.

Andrade, S. J. Family roles of Hispanic women: Stereotypes, empirical findings and implications for research. UCLA: Spanish Speaking Mental Health Research Center, 1981c. In press.

Anguiano, L. Days of the Mexican American woman. *The newsletter of NWEE,* National Women's Employment and Education, Inc., July-December 1979, *2,* 4.

Arce, A., and Torres Matrullo, C. Treatment modalities with acculturated Puerto Rican patients. In *Hispanic Report on Families and Youth.* Washington, D.C.: COSSMHO, 1980, 71-75.

Baker, G. N. Social work through an interpreter. *Social Work,* September 1981, *26,* No. 5, 391-397.

Bauman, R. Surviving stress. *American Way,* January 1980, 52-56.

Bem, S. L. Sex-role adaptability: One consequence of psychological androgyny. *Journal of Personality and Social Psychology,* 1975a, *31,* 634-643.

Bem, S. L. Androgyny vs. the tight little lives of fluffy women and chesty men. *Psychology Today,* September, 1975b, 58-62.

Benitez, J. S. The little traditions of Hispanics. *Agenda,* May/June 1980, *10,* No. 3, 30-36.

Boulette, T. R. *Determining needs and appropriate counseling approaches for Mexican American women: A comparison of therapeutic listening and behavioral rehearsal.* San Francisco: Rand E. Research Associates, 1976a. Monograph.

Boulette, T. R. Assertive training with low income Mexican American women. In M. R. Miranda (Ed.), *Psychotherapy with Spanish Speaking: Issues in Research and Service Delivery.* Monograph number 3. Los Angeles: University of California, 1976b, 67-71.

Burruel, G., and Chavez, N. Mental health outpatient centers: Relevant or irrelevant to Mexican Americans. In A. B. Tulipan, C. L. Attneave and E. Kington (Eds.), *Beyond Clinic Walls,* University, Al: University of Alabama Press, 1974.

Canino, I. A., & Canino, G. Impact of stress on the Puerto Rican family: Treatment consideration. *American Journal of Orthopsychiatry.* July 1980, *50,* No. 3, 535-541.

Carrillo, C. Directions for Chicano psychotherapy. In M. M. Casas and S. E. Keefe (Eds.), *Family and Mental Health in the Mexican American Community.* Monograph number seven, Los Angeles: The Spanish Speaking Mental Health Research Center, 1978, 125-156.

Chavez, N. Foreword. In P. P. Martin (Ed.), *La Frontera perspective: Providing mental health services to Mexican Americans.* Tucson: La Frontera Center, Inc.: 1979, xi-xix.

Chestang, L. *Character development in a hostile environment.* Occasional Paper #3. Monograph. School of Social Service Administration, Chicago. 1972.

Conference on the educational and occupational needs of Hispanic women. June 29-30, 1976, December 10-12, 1976. U. S. Dept. of Education Office of Educational Research and Improvement. National Institute of Education, September 1980.

Cotera, M. Mexicano feminism: The Chicano and the Anglo versions, a historical analysis. In M. B. Melville (Ed.), *Twice a Minority: Mexican American Women.* St. Louis: The C. V. Mosby Company, 1980, 217-234.

Cromwell, R. E., and Ruiz, R. A. The myth of macho dominance in decision making within Mexican and Chicano families. *Hispanic Journal of Behavioral Sciences.* December 1979, *1,* No. 4, 355-373.

Cruz, A. M. Biculturalism and androgyny: New perspectives for understanding Chicanos. *Research Bulletin.* Spanish Speaking Mental Health Research Center. University of California, Los Angeles. February 1977, *2*, No. 1, 1-2.

Dieppa, D., and Montiel, M. Hispanic families: An exploration. In M. Montiel (Ed.), *Hispanic Families—Critical Issues for Policy and Programs in Human Services.* COSSMHO, Washington, D. C., 1978, 1-8.

Fallis, G. V. The liberated Chicana—A struggle against tradition. *Women.* 1974, *3*, No. 4, 20-21.

Fischer, J. *Effective casework practice: An eclectic approach.* New York: McGraw-Hill, 1978.

Fitzpatrick, J. P. The Puerto Rican family. In C. H. Mindel and R. W. Habenstein (Eds.), *Ethnic Families in America: Patterns and Variations.* New York: Elsevier, 1976, 192-217.

Freese, A. S. *Understanding Stress.* Public Affairs Pamphlet no. 538, 1980.

Fried, M. Endemic stress: The psychology of resignation and the politics of scarcity. *American Journal of Orthopsychiatry.* January 1982, *52*, No. 1, 4-19.

Garcia, F. The cult of virginity. In *Conference on the educational and occupational needs of Hispanic Women.* Office of Education Research and Improvement. National Institute of Education. September 1980, 65-73.

Garcia-Bahne, B. La Chicana and the Chicano family. In R. Sanchez and R. M. Cruz (Eds.), *Essays on La Mujer.* Chicano Studies Center Publications, University of California, Los Angeles, 1977, 30-47.

Gibson, G. An approach to identification and prevention of developmental difficulties among Mexican-American children. *American Journal of Orthopsychiatry.* January 1978, *48*, No. 1, 96-113.

Gibson, R. W. Evaluation and quality control of mental health services. In E. R. Padilla and A. M. Padilla (Eds.), *Transcultural Psychiatry: An Hispanic Perspective.* Monograph number four. UCLA: Spanish Speaking Mental Health Research Center, 1977, . 13-20.

Gilbert, J. M. Extended family integration among second-generation Mexican Americans. In C. Manuel and S. E. Keefe (Eds.), *Family and Mental Health in the Mexican-American Community.* UCLA: The Spanish Speaking Mental Health Research Center, 1978, 25-48.

Gomez, E., and Becker, R. E. (Eds.), *Mexican American language and culture: Implications for helping professions.* Part I. San Antonio, Worden School of Social Service, Our Lady of the Lake University of San Antonio, 1979.

Gomez, E., and Cerda, G. *The Social Significance and Value Dimensions of Current Mexican American dialected Spanish: A Glossary for Human Service Professions.* San Antonio: Worden School of Social Service, Our Lady of the Lake University, 1976.

Gutierrez, M. E. The Latino family—Linking the past and the future. *Agenda,* January/February 1979, *9,* No. 1.

Hart, D. Enlarging the American Dream: Women. Reprinted for American Education, May 1977, 13, No. 4.

Hassell, S. S. Depression in Mexican-American Women: Implications for community mental health services. *IDRA Newsletter,* July 1980, 4-6.

Hynes, K., and Werbin, J. Group psychotherapy for Spanish-speaking women. *Psychiatric Annals,* 1977, *7,* No. 12, 52-63.

It's your turn in the sun, Hispanic Americans: Soon the biggest minority. Cover story. *Time.* October 16, 1978.

Jaramillo, M. R. How to succeed in business and remain Chicana. Keynote Address. Fourth annual MANA training conference. Washington, D. C., July 25, 1980.

Jimenez-Vazquez, R. Social issues confronting Hispanic-American women. In *Conference on the educational and occupational needs of Hispanic women.* Office of Education Research and Improvement. National Institute of Education, September 1980, 213-249.

Keefe, S. E. Why Mexican-Americans underutilize mental health clinics: Fact and fallacy.

In J. M. Casas and S. E. Keefe (Eds.), *Family and Mental Health in the Mexican American Community*, Monograph No. 7. Los Angeles: Spanish-Speaking Mental Health Research Center, 1978, 91-108.

Kline, F., Austin, W., Acosta, F. X., and Johnson, R. G. Subtle bias in the treatment of the Spanish-speaking patient. In E. R. Padilla and A. M. Padilla (Eds.), *Transcultural Psychiatry: An Hispanic Perspective,* Monograph No. 4. Los Angeles: Spanish-Speaking Research Center, 1977, 73-77.

Lara-Braud, J. The status of religion among Mexican Americans. In M. M. Mangold (Ed.), *La Causa Chicana: The Movement for Justice.* New York: Family Service Association of America, 1972, 87-94.

Lazarus, R. S. Little hassles can be hazardous to your health. *Psychology Today.* July 1981, *15,* No. 7, 58-62.

Levine, E. S., and Padilla, A. *Crossing cultures in therapy: Pluralistic counseling for Hispanics.* Monterrey, Ca.: Brooks/Cole Publishing Co., 1980.

Marrero, M. S. A letter to my mother (an attempt at communicating). *Nuestro,* February 1978, *2,* No. 2, 59.

Martinez, D. R. Protestant ministries increasing. *Agenda,* November/December 1978, *8,* No. 6, 8.

Mason, T. A discussion of the Chicano women's movement. In M. B. Melville (Ed.), *Twice a Minority: Mexican American Women.* St. Louis: The C. V. Mosby Co., 1980, 95-108.

Medina, C., and Reyes, M. R. Dilemmas of Chicano counselors. *Social Work,* November 1976, *21,* No. 6, 515-517.

Melville, M. B. Introduction. In M. B. Melville (Ed.), *Twice a Minority: Mexican American Women.* St. Louis: The C. V. Mosby Co., 1980a, 1-9.

Melville, M. B. Selective acculturation of female Mexican migrants. In M. B. Melville (Ed.), *Twice a Minority: Mexican American Women.* St. Louis: The C. V. Mosby Co., 1980b, 155-163.

Mirande, A., and Enriquez, E. *La Chicana: The Mexican American Woman.* Chicago: The University of Chicago Press, 1979.

Montiel, M. The social science myth of the Mexican American family. In O. Romano (Ed.), *Voices.* Quinto Sol Publications. 1970, 57-64.

Montiel, M. Foreword. In M. Montiel (Ed.), *Hispanic families—critical issues for policy and programs in human services.* COSSMHO, Washington, D. C., 1978, ix-x.

Moore, John R., and Andrew, Sylvia R. Mexican American cultural family assessment, San Antonio: Worden School of Social Service, Our Lady of the Lake University, mimeographed, undated.

Morales, A. The need for nontraditional mental health programs in the barrio. In J. M. Casas and S. E. Keefe (Eds.), *Family and mental health in the Mexican American community.* 1978, 125-142.

Murillo, N. The Mexican-American family. In N. N. Wagner and M. J. Haug (Eds.), *Chicanos, social and psychological perspectives.* The C. V. Mosby Co., 1971. 97-108.

Nieto, C. The Chicana and the women's rights movement. *Civil Rights Digest, a quarterly of the U.S. Commission on Civil Rights,* Spring, 1972, 36-42.

Padilla, A. M. Delivery of community mental health services to the Spanish-speaking Spanish-surnamed population. In R. Alvarez (Ed.), *Delivery of Services for Latino Community Mental Health.* Los Angeles: Spanish-Speaking Mental Health Research and Development Program, 1975.

Padilla, A. M., and Ruiz, R. A. *Latino Mental Health: A review of literature.* (DHEW Publication No. HSM 73-9143). Washington, D.C.: U.S. Government Printing Office, 1973.

Philippus, M. J. Successful and unsuccessful approaches to mental health services for an urban Hispano American Population. *Journal of Public Health,* 1971, *61,* No. 4, 820-830.

Ramirez, M., III. Recognizing and understanding diversity: Multiculturalism and the Chicano movement in psychology. In J. L. Martinez, Jr. (Ed.), *Chicano Psychology.* New York: Academic Press, 1977, 343-360.

Ramirez, R. Machismo: A bridge rather than a barrier to family and marital counseling. In P. O. Martin (Ed.), *La Frontera perspective: Providing mental health services to Mexican Americans.* Monograph number one. Tucson: La Frontera Center, Inc., 1979, 61-62.

Rendon, A. B. *Chicano manifesto.* New York: Collier Books, 1971.

Romano, I. Social science objectivity and the Chicanos. In O. Romano (Ed.), *Voices.* Quinto Sol Publications, 1973, 43-56.

Ruiz, R. A., Casas, J. M., and Padilla, A. M. *Culturally relevant behavioristic counseling.* Los Angeles: Spanish Speaking Mental Health Research Center, UCLA, Occasional Paper No. 5, 1977.

Salazar, S. Reproductive choice for Hispanas. *Agenda.* July/August, 1979, 9, No. 4.

Salazar, S. A. Women and reproductive health issues. In *Hispanic report on families and Youth.* Washington, D.C.: COSSMHO, 1980, 37-42.

Sandoval, M. The Latinization of the Catholic Church. *Agenda,* November/December, 1978, 8, No. 6, 4-8.

Senour, M. N. Psychology of the Chicana. In J. L. Martinez (Ed.), *Chicano Psychology.* New York: Academic Press, 1977, 329-342.

Solis, F. Socioeconomic and cultural conditions of migrant workers. In M. M. Mangold (Ed.), *La Causa Chicana: The Movement for Justice.* New York: Family Service Association of America, 1972, 179-191.

Szapocznik, J., and Truss, C. Intergenerational sources of role conflict in Cuban mothers. In M. Montiel (Ed.), *Hispanic families—critical issues for policy and programs in human services.* COSSMHO, Washington, D.C., 1978, 41-65.

Terrones, E. Some thoughts of a macho on the Chicana movement. *Agenda,* November/December 1977, 7, No. 6, 35-36.

Torrey, M., and Fuller, E. The irrelevancy of traditional mental health services for urban Mexican-Americans. *American Journal of Orthopsychiatry.* 1970, 40, 240-241.

Ulibarri, H. Administration of bilingual education. In *Put Research Into Education Practice.* - PREP #6-A. HEW Office of Education (Undated, mimeographed paper).

Urdaneta, M. L. Chicana use of abortion. In M. B. Melville (Ed.), *Twice a Minority: Mexican American Women.* St. Louis: The C. V. Mosby Co., 1980, 33-51.

Vaca, N. The Mexican Americans in the social sciences. *El Grito,* 1970, 4.

Vassiliou, V. G., and Vassiliou, G. Variations of the group process across cultures. *The International Journal of Group Psychotherapy,* January, 1974, XXIV, No. 1, 55-65.

Vivo, P. Voces de Hispanas: Hispanic women and their concerns. In *Hispanics and grantmakers: A special report of foundation news.* The Foundation News, 1981, 35-39.

Zinn, M. B. Chicanas: Power and control in the domestic sphere. *De Colores,* 1975a, 3, No. 1, 21-23.

Zinn, M. B. Political familism: Toward sex role equality in Chicano families. *Aztlan,* 1975b, 6, No. 1, 13-26.

Zinn, M. B. Marital roles and ethnicity: Conceptual revisions and new research directions. In *Hispanic report on families and youth.* Washington, D.C.: COSSMHO, 1980, 31-35.

Black Women:
A Tradition of Self-Reliant Strength

Christine Renee Robinson

Black women, and the complexity of our lives, must be included in the development of any psychological theory of women. As I read current theories, books or articles on the psychology of women or feminist therapy, I am constantly struck by the omissions. Pertinent theory on Black women's psychological development is rarely included. What has been widely available are graphic descriptions of the inherent pathologies of Black women and Black families (Thomas & Sillen, 1972). Only recently have Black and minority journals, anthologies, and texts begun to include an increasing number of articles focusing specifically on Black women. Psychological and social theories must be based on the sociohistorical reality of a people and the richness of their cultural heritage.

When a knowledge and acceptance of these realities are developed in theory and practice, social scientists, researchers, or therapists will be able to work effectively with Black women. Mental health practitioners who aspire to humanist ideals are caught up in the sexist and racist ideologies of the dominant culture. They participate in perpetuating the oppressive myths by labelling clients, or encouraging them to accept the racist, sexist and pathologizing practices and views of society. Effective therapy should encourage the individual to develop, utilize, and value inner strengths, regardless of societal norms.

Black women, the most disadvantaged group in the United States, as evidenced by their unenviable occupational, educa-

The author is a graduate of Vassar College. She is a Program Evaluation Specialist, New York State Office of Mental Health, completing her MS in Developmental Psychology at Cornell University.

135

tional, employment, income, and male-availability levels, have been "messed-over" by distorters of reality. . .This distortion successfully continues the oppression of Black women and indirectly Black men, thereby masking the real racist and sexist culprits (Jackson, 1973, p. 254).

The double bind of living in a racist and sexist society has placed Black women in an extremely difficult position. Black women are the poorest paid workers (Olmedo & Parron, 1981), have shorter life expectancies, higher infant mortality rates, are more likely to contract stress-related diseases (Jackson, 1973), are more likely to be diagnosed as having a chronic rather than an acute mental illness, and are most likely to be institutionalized for mental illness (Smith, 1981). Reports from the 1975 census reveal that there are 9.2% more Black females than Black males, making a plurality of female-headed households a certainty (Copeland, 1982). The conditions under which most Black women live have been harsh. Furthermore, our remarkable strengths and coping abilities have been purposely distorted by social scientists.

Black women, due to economic necessity, have always worked to support themselves and their families. We have been forced by society, oppression, our position, and our tradition to be responsible for the economic, social, and physical survival of our families and communities, regardless of socioeconomic status, age, geographic location, or educational attainment. Our adaptability to varied roles, while transcending societal barriers, illustrates significant coping abilities.

The mass movement of White women into the labor force during the 1970s forced women and society to review their perceptions of appropriate sex roles, raising "new concerns" in the field of mental health. For centuries, Black women have been dealing creatively with these same concerns: role adaptability, division of household chores, working wives/mothers, sexual harassment/abuse, and coping with stressful situations. As Filomina Steady (1981) states, Black women are the "original feminists."

Black women in the society are the only ethnic or radical group which has had the opportunity to be women. By this I simply mean that much of the current focus on being liberated from the constraints and protectiveness of the society which is proposed by women's liberation groups has never applied to Black women, and in that sense, we have always been "free," and able to develop as individuals even under the most harsh circumstances. This freedom, as well as the tremendous hardships from which Black women suffered, allowed for the development of a personality that is rarely described in the scholarly journals for its obstinate strength and ability to survive. Neither is its peculiar humanistic character and quiet courage viewed as the epitome of what the American model of Femininity should be. (Joyce Ladner, 1972, p. 280).

The Black woman embodies the essence of psychological androgyny, though she has not been so described by others. The so-called "masculine" traits of self-reliance, independence, assertiveness, and strength are inherent characteristics of Black women which are passed on to Black girls at a very early age. Although these traits are considered appropriate when displayed by men, and are the very traits which feminists strive to adopt, these traits are perceived as extremely threatening by Whites when developed and exhibited by Black women.

The Black woman has devised a coping strategy to care for herself and her family, following a tradition of self-reliance and independence. However, this strategy has been labelled by social scientists as pathological, inappropriate, even detrimental to the family she seeks to protect. Her strength is viewed as "dominating" and "castrating," and *she* is blamed for the scars oppression has left upon her people.

Literature, movies, and advertisements, have consistently portrayed Black women in a stereotypical derogatory manner, as "Mammy," "Sapphire," or "Whore." Social science has diagnosed Black females as being intellectually inferior, sexually promiscuous, and possessing a "dominating character" (Moynihan, 1965). This female dominance or "matriarchal character" of the Black family is supposedly responsible for such varied ills as juvenile delinquency, the unemployment of Black men, lower educational attainment of Black men, and low I.Q. scores (Pettigrew, 1964). Works by Billingsley (1969), Cade (1970), Jackson (1973), Simms-Brown (1982), Staples (1970, 1973), Willie (1981), vehemently refute Moynihan's 1965 mis-interpretation of the dynamics within the Black family. Ironically, Black families have been labelled in this way because our familial structure is not "traditionally patriarchal." Although society seems to be currently more receptive to differing family structures, I have seen no retraction of these detrimental theories.

It is both racist and sexist to view the strengths of Black women as pathological, instead of recognizing and commending the effective coping mechanisms that have been developed out of necessity, and are perpetuated due to their functional value. The implications, origins and sociohistorical significance of Black women's self-reliance must be recognized and understood by the psychological, therapeutic, and feminist community. These women are indeed androgynous and have been feminists for centuries.

> From that time (Emancipation) to the present day, each generation of women, following in the footsteps of their mothers, has borne a large share of the support of the younger generation (Frazier, 1939, p. 103).

The legacy, from our mothers and grandmothers, is an inherent part of our community and culture. The cross-cultural tradition, which encompasses all women of African descent within the African diaspora, is a profound and meaningful one. Our African foremothers are the bearers of this tradition. A Pan-African perspective on the development of feminine roles in society requires that one understand the etiology, the collective-consciousness.

African women were the backbone of their traditional societies, assuming a large economic responsibility. They were respected for the work performed and for the autonomous position they occupied within society. Traditionally sex roles were egalitarian, women and men shared responsibility for tasks to be accomplished, female subordination was not an issue. African societies were primarily agricultural economies in which women occupied a central role as farmers, traders, home-builders, homemakers, and childcare providers. They were active in community politics and tribal affairs (Steady, 1981).

The origin of this respect for women and their independent roles can be found in several traditional African religions. The Egyptian Queen Mother, Hathor, Goddess of Creation, gave birth to the universe and established the traditions of her people. In Islam, Allat was the mother of Allah. In Northeast Africa, Mawu, the Creator-Goddess, made the earth and created humanity. Ala is the earth mother of Nigeria. Several other goddesses hold central positions in African religions, Nut, Ishtar, Mella, Bomu Rambi. The Bantu goddess Songi as the protector of women supports the ownership of lands, homes, and property by women, abhors any abusive treatment of women, and ensures that men treat women respectfully (Stone, 1980; Monaghan, 1981).

African religion, culture, and social structure accentuate the traits of courage, independence, strength, and perseverance. Our foremothers are women who strove to cultivate these traits within an established tradition as self-reliant workers, and respected egalitarian family and community members.[1] Without the fortitude of these essential traits, Black women would not have survived the grueling and dehumanizing years of slavery.

The debasing role of laborer and breeder during slavery, served to degrade the Black woman in the minds of Whites, undermine her sense of self, and thoroughly exploit her body. She was bought and sold, she worked in the fields alongside the men, her rape and beatings were sanctioned and encouraged, and her children were frequently sold. Her femininity was ignored; no differential treatment was given to the slave woman. Regardless of pregnancy or age, she performed the same exhausting work as slave men, and was beaten as severely (Davis, 1981). Furthermore, Black womanhood was defiled by rampant sexual abuse.

·The Black woman's victimization can be illustrated no more vividly than in her history of sexual abuse. She was raped often, and her rape was sanctioned. If current idealized values of femininity are used as a standard for comparison, the Black woman falls totally outside the boundaries. The White woman was portrayed as virtuous, an object of chivalry, her sexuality was guarded and treasured. The Black woman's sexuality was abused and defiled as she confronted the daily reality of physical and psychological rape. American society tried very hard to destroy her sense of integrity, the core of her sense of self-worth. Yet, she managed to maintain a semblance of family. Since Black men were forbidden to protect their families by slaveowners, and slave marriages were not recognized, the mother-child bond remained the essential family link, as long as the child was not sold. Some slave mothers killed their children rather than see them sold into slavery (Ladner, 1981). Black women had few expectations of economic dependence upon

---

[1]With the advent of capitalism, the role of women in Africa was forced to change. The imposition of European values upon African culture and the introduction of Western religion brought a marked change to the expected role of women in society (Steady, 1981).

their men. They did not expect a protected or symbiotic existence. Their legacy had been of women and men working alongside each other, thus making sex roles more egalitarian (Millham & Smith, 1981). E. Franklin Frazier (1939) states, "Emancipation tended to confirm in many cases the spirit of self-sufficiency slavery had taught."

The Black Women's Club Movement of the late 1800s and earlier 1900s was organized as a response to lynching, and was responsible for the first organized protest against sexual abuse of women (Davis, 1981). The National Association of Colored Women and the National Council of Negro Women strove to ennoble Black women and men, to address the needs of the Black community, to protest lynching, sexual abuse of women, and conditions in prisons, to fight for unionization, and to address all oppressive conditions (Davis, 1981).

Historically Black women have always been at the forefront of the struggle for human rights: Harriet Tubman, Ida B. Wells, Mary Church Terrell, Mary McLeod Bethune, Shirley Chisholm, Angela Davis, the list goes on. Frequently Black women have been the initiating and instigating force that challenged and confronted social issues (Murray, 1975). Their work has been a life's work, a race's work, a culture's work. Sojourner Truth's eloquent statement made at the Women's Rights Convention in Akron, Ohio in 1852 is as timely today as it was when it was first given:

Ain't I A Woman?

That man over there say
  a woman needs to be helped into carriages
and lifted over ditches
  and to have the best place everywhere.
Nobody ever helped me into carriages
  or over mud puddles
    or gives me a best place. . .
Ain't I a woman?
  Look at me
Look at my arm!
  I have plowed and planted
and gathered into barns
  and no man could head me. . .
And ain't I a woman?

I could work as much
and eat as much as a man—
when I could get it—
and bear the lash as well
and ain't I a woman?
I have borne 13 children
and seen most all sold into slavery
and when I cried out a mother's grief
none but Jesus heard me. . .
and ain't I a woman?
That little man in black there say
a woman can't have as much rights as a man
cause Christ wasn't a woman
Where did your Christ come from?
From God and a woman!
Man had nothing to do with him!
If the first woman God ever made
Was strong enough to turn the world
upside down, all alone
together women ought to be able to turn it
rightside up again.

The collective spirit of togetherness, sharing strength and mutual support, is a tradition within the Black community. The traditional extended family still exists in practice and ideology. A strong affiliation binds Black women, and a natural reaching out to others occurs in the family itself and in the larger community. College students form peer groups quite akin to extended families (Carroll, 1981). The church, the hairdresser, and the "juke-joint" have become the institutions through which one seeks support, guidance, and comfort. The Black woman's self-worth is measured by her likeness to other Black women in the community (Meyers, 1975). It is frequently the Black women who move from their established community, or find themselves without a sense of "belongingness," who seek help from the formal mental health services.

Women and therapists must confront their own racism and biases. Societal influences have taught us to embrace, believe, and act on theories which are erroneous. We cannot speak of a psychology of women if frameworks and perspectives are applicable only to middle-class, professional, or White women. We have much to learn from a woman in the poorest Black community, or one who succeeds despite incredible stress. Though her reality may be very different from one's own, her voice must be heard. The value of Black culture and the tradition of strengths can no longer be negated.

The literature of the feminist movement emphasizes certain factions, but lacks a holistic view. We must recognize the centrality of the issue of oppression, regardless of its origin, be it race, class, or sex. Jean Baker Miller (1976) addresses the issue of oppression in the first chapter of *Toward a New Psychology of Women*. Her discussion of "Domination-Subordination" can be applied to issues of sexism, racism, and classism in society. As we look at our sisters, let us look at all of them and not lose sight of the central issue of oppression. Black women are very familiar with oppression. We have been coping with it for centuries.

Black women have repeatedly seen their lives defined by White or male values. Being different from both of these groups, the Black woman is often seen as pathological. The history of degradation and disparity in traditional social services would make any Black woman wary of mental health services. Black women have traditionally been denied equal access to treatment (Smith, 1981). Mental health services are usually not located in Black neighborhoods. Blacks are not seen as good therapy candidates, for the circumstances affecting their lives are not fully understood by professionals. The issue of race is frequently not a problem to the Black client, but a problem to the therapist (Thomas & Sillen, 1972). We as Black women must continue to develop our own theories, realistic practical theories, which encompass the unique Black experience. Janice Porter Gump, Harriette McAdoo, Patricia Bell Scott, Michelene Malson, Elizabeth Higginbotham, Beverly Guy-Sheftall, Lena Wright Myers, Gloria Joseph, Cheryl Gilkes, and many others have published significant works specifically addressing psychological issues of Black women. We are, and must continue to define ourselves.

In the formation of psychological theory, Black women's literary and artistic expression must also be considered. The art, music, dance, and literature of a people is the essence of their soul, the mirror of reality. *The Third Life of Grange Copeland* (1975) by Alice Walker is a far more profound and sensitive analysis of the nature of a battering relationship than any case study I have ever read. Toni Morrison and Maya Angelou both address issues of sexual abuse of children and the surrounding family dynamics. The psychological reality of black women, expressed in poetry, blues lyrics, and novels, contains more sociohistorical data than is currently to be found in any psychology text.

Mary Helen Washington (1981), an English professor, editor, and author, describes the "divided self" within Black women: this is the nature of the dichotomy between our reality, our talents, and our dreams. Washington characterizes the "suspended woman," severely limited in her options, destroyed by pain, pressure, and violence; the "assimilated woman," one who strives to assimilate into the mainstream culture, alienated from her roots and culture; and the "emergent woman" one with a new awareness, who confronts and sorts out the issues of her reality. Washington's work presents the nucleus of a psychological theory of Black women.

Black women through religion, culture, and our very being have a history of self-reliant feminism. We are a product of our environment and history. We have been taught survival skills, and we possess great strength as a people. The life experiences of Black women are treasures. This is, and has been our reality, life, culture, history, experience, our legacy. We recognize and celebrate our independence and strength.

REFERENCES

Angelou, M. *I Know Why The Caged Bird Sings.* New York: Bantam Books, 1969.

Billingsley, A. *Black Families in White America.* Englewood Cliffs: Prentice Hall, 1969.

Cade, T. *The Black Woman.* New York: New American Library, 1970.

Carroll, C. Three's a Crowd: The Dilemma of the Black Woman In Higher Education. In P. Scott, B. Smith, G. Hull (Eds.), *But Some of Us Are Brave.* Old Westbury: Feminist Press, 1981.

Copeland, E. Oppressed Conditions and the Mental Health Needs of Low Income Black Women: Barrier to Services, Strategies for Change. *Women & Therapy,* Spring 1982, *1* (1), p. 13-26.

Davis, A. *Women, Race, and Class.* New York: Random House, 1981.

Frazier, E. *The Negro Family in the United States.* Chicago: University of Chicago Press, 1939.

Jackson, J. Black Women in a Racist Society. In C. Willie, B. Kramer, B. Brown (Eds.), *Racism and Mental Health.* Pittsburgh: University of Pittsburgh Press, 1973.

Ladner, J. Racism and Tradition: Black Womanhood in Historical Perspective. In F. Steady (Ed.), *The Black Woman Cross-Culturally,* Cambridge: Schenkman Publ. 1981.

Ladner, J. *Tomorrow's Tomorrow.* Garden City: Anchor Books, 1972.

Miller, J. B. *Toward A New Psychology of Women.* Boston: Beacon Press, 1976.

Millham, J., & Smith, L. Sex-role Differentiation Among Black and White Americans: A Comparative Study. *Journal of Black Psychology,* February 1981, *1,* p. 77-90.

Monaghan, P. *Book of Goddesses and Heroines.* New York: E. P. Dutton Press, 1981.

Morrison, T. *The Bluest Eye.* New York: Holt, Rinehart, and Winston, 1970.

Moynihan, D. The Negro Family: *The Case for National Action.* Washington, D.C.: U.S. Government Printing Office, 1965.

Murray, P. The Liberation of Black Women. In J. Freeman (Ed.), *Women: A Feminist Perspective.* Palo Alto: Mayfield Pub. 1975.

Myers, L. Black Women and Self-Esteem. In Millman and Kanter (Eds.), *Another Voice.* Garden City: Anchor Press, 1975.

Olmedo, E., & Parron, D. Mental Health of Minority Women. *Professional Psychology,* February 1981, *12,* pp. 103-111.

Pettigrew, T. *A Profile of the Negro American.* Princeton: Van Nostrand, 1964.

Scott, P., Smith, B., & Hull, G. *But Some Of Us Are Brave.* Old Westbury: Feminist Press, 1981.

Simms-Brown, R. The Female in the Black Family: Dominant Mate or Helpmate. *Journal of Black Psychology, 9,* pp. 45-55.

Smith, E. Mental Health and Service Delivery Systems for Black Women. *Journal of Black Studies,* December 1981, *12,* pp. 126-141.

Staples, R. *The Black Woman in America.* Chicago: Nelson Hall Pub. 1973.

Steady, F. *The Black Woman Cross-Culturally.* Cambridge: Schenkman Pub. 1981.

Stone, M. *Ancient Mirrors of Womanhood* (Vol. 1) New York: New Sibylline Books, 1980.

Truth, S. Ain't I A Woman? In E. Stetson (ed.), *Black Sister.* Bloomington: Indiana Univ. Press, 1981.

Thomas, A., & Sillen, S. *Racism and Psychiatry,* New York: Brunner Mazel, 1972.

Walker, A. *The Third Life of Grange Copeland.* New York: Harcourt, Brace, Jovanovich, 1970.

Washington, M. H. Teaching Black-Eyed Susans An Approach to the Study of Black Women Writers, in P. Scott, B. Smith, G. Hull (eds.), *But Some Of Us Are Brave.* Old Westbury: Feminist Press, 1981.

Willie, C. Dominance in the Family: The Black and White Experience. *Journal of Black Psychology,* February 1981, *7,* pp. 91-97.

A Lesbian Perspective

Jane Mara

We are in a time of crisis on Earth today: will the human species survive or will we become extinct? Like all crises this one provides us with the opportunity to grow and to expand to our farthest limits and beyond, to evolve to a new and higher consciousness.

Our impetus is twofold: first, we dread the possible extinction of the species if we don't change. Second, human life desires to fulfill its promise, the promise we each feel at some time in our hearts that life on Earth could be one of peace and joy, of cooperation and harmony. These are the forces of fear and love, of repulsion and attraction, the two primary forces which operate in human beings on Earth.

Patriarchy, the culture which dominates the Earth today, is founded on fear and rules by force, that is, some humans hold power over others. When we are in fear we hand over our power to those who threaten us. Being afraid we act in ways based not on our own inner desires but on orders from others. In so doing we lose touch with ourselves; our strengths and self-respect diminish. Our special human qualities and gifts, our creativeness and ingenuity, our powers of imagination and intuition are lost and we languish as a species on the brink of extinction entirely of our own making.

If we are to survive we must leave behind this fear-based reality and the consciousness on which it is built and move forward, creating a new reality founded on a new consciousness, one based on attraction rather than fear. Patriarchy, by definition, is founded on a male view of the world. It is time now to balance this male domination of consciousness with an equal measure of female consciousness. With such a balance comes the possibility of a creative and powerful synthesis evolving into yet a third consciousness, one

---

The author was a lesbian-feminist psychotherapist and co-founder of the Women's Growth and Therapy Center Collective in Washington, D.C. She is now living in Ireland, writing a fantasy-vision of a possible future.

which can enable us to create what has been glimpsed only in dreams and visions, a world in which human beings live in harmony with each other and with all the inhabitants and forces of our home, the Earth.

A woman who is a lesbian, because of the unique experiences which are hers, has the opportunity to learn and comprehend two processes which are needed by the human species today: one, shifting from a fear-based reality to one founded on love or attraction, and two, creating a new reality. This knowledge born from and infused with female consciousness is therefore particularly valuable at this time.

This article is about the experiences which are special to lesbians, emphasizing the opportunities they offer to evolve a new consciousness and to create a new reality. It is my hope that it will help lesbians who are involved in this journey become conscious of the evolutionary potentialities inherent in their daily lives, help those in the mental health field become aware of these potentialities, and that it will thus counteract the insidious and still popular notion that to be lesbian is in some ways a sin or a tragedy.

This article is based on the experiences and thoughts of many lesbians including myself. I am white and middle-class, and the paper thus reflects this perspective.*

There are five major experiences which lesbians encounter: being a womon** sexually loving wimmin—loving those like one's self; being taboo; coming out; detaching from the patriarchy; and creating an alternative reality.

BEING A WOMON SEXUALLY LOVING WIMMIN— LOVING THOSE LIKE ONE'S SELF

The lesbian's journey starts here, making love with a womon. She experiences her own body in relation to another womon's body, familiar because of its similarity to her own—soft, with breasts, hips, vulva, clitoris, and vagina. In loving this other woman's body she comes to love her own on the profound and unconsciousness

---

*For balance from wimmin of color and various classes see: Moraga, C., and Anzaldua, G. (Eds.), *This bridge called my back: writings of radical women of color*. Watertown, Mass., Persephone Press, 1981, and Stanley, P., and Wolfe, S. J. (Eds.), *The coming out stories*, Watertown, Mass., Persephone Press, 1980.

**The spelling womon or wimmin comes, as far as I know, from early lesbian feminist writing as wimmin began to create a reality independent of men.

level of the body, for in loving another womon she is also loving herself. There is a female fullness in this knowledge that is different from that which comes through loving a man's body, for it comes through sameness not difference. This knowledge of self is at the very core of being.

The intimate relationship which develops with a womon is also different from that with a man. Some of this difference is culture based because of sex-role stereotyping. Since wimmin are encouraged in our nurturing, caring, emotional and vulnerable natures, our capacity for intimacy is very deep. The intimacy which develops between wimmin can more easily be mutually emotional, affectionate, and nurturing than intimacy in heterosexual relationships. Two wimmin can be more spontaneously themselves because of the lack of sex-role stereotyping of behavior between wimmin in intimate sexual relationships. This is especially true concerning power, and lesbians have the opportunity to learn to share power equally in a way that is extraordinarily satisfying and conducive to intimacy.

Lesbian lovemaking then, leads to a knowledge of self as a womon on the conscious level of relationship and the unconscious level of the body as she is drawn into being herself in an entirely female context.

> I was quite ambivalent about my body before I became a lesbian. I think it was a reaction to the way wimmin's bodies are treated in the patriarchy; dressed up, shaved, sanitized, controlled, raped and generally objectified. I bought it all and objectified my own body from myself. Then, making love with a womon—it was so amazing. When my hands touched her body, so soft, amazingly soft, it was as if I was touching my own body and I became real to myself for the first time in my life. The more I love her body the more I love my own. In all the years I slept with men I never had anything like this experience.

> The first time I was sexual with a womon something in my very center opened up, something I had denied all my life. I sat on the bed and wept. I was coming home.

> When I finally got over the shock and surprise of how easy and wonderful it was, something happened that I still can't explain exactly but it is as though my *body* loves her *body* in a way that is separate from our personalities, from our loving

each other as people. It isn't just sexual desire either, it seems deeper than that, older than that. It has to do with the mutual identification that is possible between two wimmin making love, being both the giver and receiver at the same time, my whole being in my body and in hers as well. It is a profound spiritual experience.

Being Taboo

To be lesbian is to be taboo. This is a fact in most cultures of the world and is certainly true of the USA today. The particular nature of the taboo may vary with race, class, age, and culture but the essential fact of being taboo remains. Even with the advent of the Women's Movement and the Gay Liberation Movement the taboo still prevails; there are few lesbians who do not have to contend with it to some extent. The popular viewpoint remains: a lesbian is "sick," "perverted," or "evil," a womon to be feared, pitied, punished, cured, ostracized, or locked away.

Being taboo is a fearsome business for the threatened reprisals are awesome: personal and institutional rejection; loss of children, job, housing, family friends; ridicule; physical punishment; incarceration; death. When a lesbian faces these threats and decides that the actualizing of her own inclinations is worth the potential reprisals, she is taking a courageous step which increases her self-respect. It is a step taken forward toward something she loves (other wimmin and herself) and a step away from living out of fear. It is a step grounded in her own experience of herself and not based on the judgements of others.

> Taboo? In my state it's illegal to be a lesbian. How am I going to get custody of my children if I'm illegal because of my very nature? Yet I can't deny myself who I am, can I? I'm young and alive and very sexual. I could move to another state but this is my home. I love it here. It's a damned hard life pretending not to be in love, pretending to have boyfriends, pretending to my children—that's the worst. I'm afraid they'll tell their father and who knows what he'd do with that information? Yet it's no good lying to my own children. I'm not sure what I'll do but I have to do something. I have to be able to be real with my children even if it means not having custody. Pretending is worse—then we are all living paper-doll lives.

I was so frightened when I looked at her and felt my body respond. What was I, one of those horrid "dykes"? Could people see? Would I be kicked out of school? I knew what happened to girls like that—they disappeared and were never seen again. Yet I couldn't deny it, my body was going wild. I avoided her for months, avoided my body too, until eventually I couldn't deny it anymore. Once we made love, the whole world changed. I knew inside that I'd found myself. This great peace descended on me. I kept it a secret, though, for years. I may have accepted myself and her but I wasn't ready for the rejection that I knew would follow if I told my family. For years I lived a double life.

Coming Out

The next step in this lesbian's journey is declaring that she is a lesbian. Many wimmin who are sexual with other wimmin never make this statement even to themselves and some make it to themselves and their lovers but go no further. Most lesbians, however, come out to some extent in our wider lives; to parents, children, friends, co-workers; where we work, play, and live. Lesbians continually face coming out as new people come into our lives, as our surroundings change and as we decide to extend our declaration of self further into the world. Coming out always takes courage for we never know what the response of the other will be. (One way for a heterosexual person to understand this process is to close your eyes and see yourself telling someone in your life that you are a homosexual.)

Coming out leads to many new awarenesses. There is the awareness of her own courage. There is the awareness of being loved, respected, cared for regardless of her lesbianism; this is reassuring and validating. There is the awareness that she is loved, respected, cared for conditionally and by being lesbian she has broken the conditions. This is usually hard and painful. Sometimes it is freeing for when she realizes that the love or respect was dependent on being "normal" or heterosexual she can be freed of the burden of such a relationship. This is often true of relationships with parents and can take many years to work through.

Coming out frequently leads to changes in a lesbian's life. When she comes out at home, school or work the atmosphere around her often changes. Other lesbians come out as well, homophobia becomes more or less evident. People treat her differently, with more or less respect, more or less care, more or less hostility. Interpersonal relationships become more or less comfortable, more or less intimate.

The consequences of coming out may cause a lesbian to change aspects of her life, leave school, change jobs, find a new place to live, or continue where she is with a new depth in her relationships or perhaps a new tension.

Not coming out leads to the necessity of containment, living a private life and sometimes a double life. Not coming out makes the boundaries between herself and those who don't know quite clear. Not coming out results in some sort of compromise with the world around her—silence and secrecy in exchange for the rewards of acceptance by the culture.

Most lesbians live with both these experiences for there are very few of us who are comfortable enough to come out completely in our lives.

> I was terrified of coming out to my parents. I was sure they would disown me. And I wasn't far from wrong. They stopped asking me anything about my personal life, seemed embarrassed by my very presence and lied about me to their friends and relatives. I was devastated at first and sorry I'd told them, but evading their questions had just become too damned difficult and painful. In the long run this was exactly what I needed. I had been very dependent on them and I had to realize that it is my life to live regardless of their support or approval. Once that finally sunk in I felt really free and made all sorts of important changes in my life, and today I'm much more the person I want to be.

> Coming out to my parents was amazing. I told them how happy I was to finally find someone I could truly and deeply love and with whom I felt free to be myself. It all had to do with loving a woman. And they were so delighted for me. I had been mildly depressed for years; they said they could see the change in me, saw parts of me reappearing which seemed to have been lost years ago. I felt free and happy after I told them.

> It was a choice. Keep working at the job pretending to be a heterosexual, come out, or quit. I was sick of pretending and

too scared to quit, so I came out. Telling people I was gay
didn't get me fired, but it didn't get me any friends either. I
was tolerated, that's the word for it, tolerated. This was worse
than before so I finally got up the courage to quit. After coming out I was much stronger and sure of myself, even though
no one there put out an iota of positive energy toward me or
gave me any support, it was like I became invisible.

I'm much happier in my life now—working at something
that is relevant to me. From the outside my life seems much
more tenuous than it was before but inside I'm much stronger.
And I'm free to really be myself, as a lesbian, wherever I am.

The attraction to freedom at some point outweighs the fears of
risking, and the desire for more freedom becomes the underlying
force in the lesbians' life.

Becoming Detached from the Patriarchy

The patriarchy is based on a lot of foolish notions and for
some reason I thought I was crazy because they didn't make
sense to me so I learned to keep my big mouth shut and tried to
find a life for myself within its boundaries. But still all these
things rankled. For example, men are superior to women and
children. Or the Earth is here to be exploited by humans and
not for Her own existence and purpose. Or ''God'' is the Great
Father in the Sky who knows better than I what I should do and
should learn to obey ''Him'' and those who speak for ''Him''
even when it goes against my own inner feelings. Or that war
makes sense. Or that people get more done through competition than cooperation. Or that the men who make the laws are
privy to some kind of wisdom whereby they can judge what is
right or wrong for other people. Or that violence is a way of
life. Or that rape even exists.

The one that tipped me over the edge, though, was the one
that said it was WRONG to have sex with someone of the same
sex. Oh, I believed that was true along with the rest, but finally
my body's voice got louder and more insistent even than all
these teachings that had been drummed into me and I took a
huge risk and went to bed with a womon. That did it. It was so
wonderful, so clearly right for me, that I took a look at everything else I'd been told, piece by piece, and threw them on the

rubbish heap right next to any sense I had that to make love with a womon is wrong. Goodbye patriarchy, hello ME.

The attraction to these freedoms; the freedom to be one's self to act on one's own inner promptings, to pursue what is in one's own mind and heart, to follow one's own beliefs can influence lesbians to let go of the reality of the patriarchy and create one of our own. Detaching is a frightening undertaking, especially when the new reality is not envisioned or created.

When lesbians move through this void and experience the loneliness that ensues, we do so because the attraction of freedom is stronger than the fears of loss, loneliness or retribution. Our courage is called again to the fore and our strengths deepen as we realize we have a choice about our lives. We learn we can choose to live in and collude with the patriarchy's creation of reality, thus strengthening and enforcing it, or we can choose to leave it behind and create a reality which nurtures and sustains us as wimmin, as lesbians individually and collectively.

In recognizing this choice we learn that we are utterly responsible for our own lives. We learn that blame is futile, a waste of time and energy, and that to blame is to stay attached. We learn instead to be angry and to use our anger to free ourselves of the patriarchy's grip—to say NO! We learn to move on.

> I languished for years in my marriage, being who I thought I "should" be, doing what I thought I was "supposed to" do and scared to death to pay attention to the voice inside of me that was screaming, "GET ME OUT OF HERE."
>
> It took the women's movement for me to see that I had options. That I had a choice. What a revelation! Of course, then I had to be responsible for the consequences of my decision. One thing about being a housewife, I could always blame everything on my husband, and that's what I did, blame, blame, blame. I blamed him for my unhappiness because I didn't have the courage to say NO to the life I was living, I was caught in a vise and couldn't move. Everything scared me— being on my own, being "queer," being angry, being rejected by my parents if I got divorced and broke up the family. Most of all I was scared of being responsible for my own life.
>
> And there's the irony because I was responsible all along, I

just didn't see it. I had chosen the marriage, I had chosen not to listen to my own voice, to swallow my anger, to act out of rear. It took two years in therapy to see this but when I finally did, I can't tell you how relieved I felt. Because being responsible meant being free! Suddenly I could be who I am; for starters I became a dyke.

Now I see that I have a choice in everything I do in my life and every time I act based on what I believe I'm helping to make it real. Having detached from my marriage I began detaching from other aspects of the patriarchy. Next came their newspapers, magazines, t.v. and films. Their version of reality is too destructive and fear producing; it's distorted from my point of view. I'm still somewhere in the middle of course, patriarchy is too omnipresent to completely avoid (I still pay taxes for example), but the more I let go the more comfortable I am and the more energy there is for creating a new world!

I knew I was different when I was very young but I didn't know why. I also knew that "different" could be "crazy" and "crazy" was dangerous. So I stopped thinking "crazy." I stopped thinking. Then, when I came out as a lesbian and realized how much I'd been lied to I began to think again, began to believe what I saw. All the inner beliefs I'd denied, my sense of reincarnation, memories of past lives, not wanting to eat animals, sensing the life force (they call it God) within me, my sense of life beyond this planet, my awareness of unrecognized powers—all this came flooding back to me in a rush. I was almost in shock for awhile it was so strong.

Then as I met other wimmin my sense of myself was validated and encouraged for they were having similar experiences, we were all saying "me too, me too," and then we all KNEW we weren't crazy.

Letting go of the patriarchal ways of thinking left an empty space into which came spiritual illumination. Becoming part of a wimmin's spirituality group and sharing this light with other lesbians is a profound experience. This sharing of energy and power takes me beyond my ego into an energy beyond. It is an energy we are learning to use and share, full of power, creativity and wisdom. It is an ancient wisdom we are tapping into, one repressed and denied out of fear (how many wimmin raped, how many wimmin burned?). As we unearth it from within ourselves and from herstory we have a potent force to use and trust. With it we can create our future.

CREATING A NEW REALITY

Moving from a patriarchal world into the lesbian world is changing realities. The lesbian world has been developing more and more openly since the beginning of the present wave of feminism. A lesbian can live her life largely within this world, especially in big cities and in rural pockets of the United States.

Lesbians: make and listen to lesbian music; we write, publish and read lesbian literature, journals, and newspapers; we organize and attend lesbian conferences, music festivals, art shows, concerts, political activities; we belong to lesbian support groups focusing on issues of concern to lesbians such as racism, classism, alcoholism, monogamy/open relationships, jealousy, lesbian motherhood, being a lesbian of a particular race, color or religion; being a lesbian in business, in academia, in the government, in high school. We learn self-defense, self-help, psychic expansion, political awareness, motorcycle maintenance, poetry making, herbal and wholistic healing, co-counseling, and lesbian herstory. Lesbians consult lesbian doctors, lawyers, accountants, dentists and healers. We eat in lesbian restaurants, drink and dance in lesbian bars, holiday at lesbian hotels, buy lesbian-made products in lesbian-owned and run shops, participate in lesbian spiritual groups, live in lesbian households and group houses, work and live on lesbian land, organize against sexism and oppression of all kinds including nuclear proliferation; lesbians go to jail with lesbians. As we do all these things we work for and share our visions of a world which will sustain and nourish us individually and collectively.

There are numerous differences between this world and the patriarchy but the central one is the way power is defined and used. In patriarchy power means power over another; it is this that breeds all oppression. In the female-centered lesbian reality power comes from within. It is the power of centeredness within oneself, not the power of aggression and oppression. In groups it is created by the circle. There is no hierarchy, no division between leader and follower. In sharing power every womon enpowered increases the power to each and all of us.

It is a revelation to experience shared power for the first time. It is a loss of Ego and a joining with a much greater energy. It depends on trust. It is difficult to learn new ways in such a non-trustful, ego-bound culture as the patriarchy. Lesbian/feminist collectives fold all too often but all the time we're learning. I often wonder if people with patriarchal consciousness would be attracted to shared power if they could experience it. Would they give up the power-over motif on their own—change their consciousness because it's in their own best interest? It seems the only way we will survive without a holocaust of some sort to clean us out. Again and again it comes down to consciousness and choice.

Lesbians' knowledge of power comes from experience; our desire for wimmin comes from our cores and as we chose to follow it we learn that acting from the center is the only true act and that in that act lies power. Joining with other lesbians we learn that the combined energy of many wimmin acting from their centers increases geometrically. Detaching from the patriarchy we discover the deep and sure knowledge that we create our own reality. Taking that responsibility and power seriously we endeavor with our minds, bodies, hearts and souls to create a world where we, and every human being, can fulfill the promise of becoming.

NEW STRATEGIES
IN FEMINIST THERAPY

In this final section, we offer new strategies for responding to the issues raised by women. Feminist therapy is committed to providing women with experiences and tools with which they can create new options and possibilities for themselves. New models of therapy emerge that recognize the relationship between the personal and the political and offer new responses to overt and covert victimization and oppression.

Sue Kirk introduces a problem-solving group model that teaches women to identify the personal, political, and structural aspects of their lives. Flora Colao and Miriam Hunt urge therapists to discard previously learned victim blaming approaches and attitudes in treating survivors of sexual abuse, replacing these with more helpful interventions learned from grassroots feminist rape crisis workers. Joan Hamerman Robbins and Rachel Josefowitz Siegel focus on different aspects of the therapist's own process of change, introducing a feminist awareness of accumulated inequalities into the work with couples.

These new feminist strategies are not limited to therapy. They expand to include the kind of legal advocacy and woman centered research we find in Terrie Lyons' paper, as well as the new structures and models for womens' groups in non-therapy settings depicted by Janette Faulkner, Sue Kirk, Janet O'Hare and Katy Taylor.

The strategies are based on the same feminist principles that have been stated in earlier chapters; respect for the client's own definition of her values and her experiences, an egalitarian, nonjudgmental helping relationship, and an awareness of the conflict between early conditioning and present ambitions. We reaffirm the importance of valuing all aspects of the client's personality and coping patterns, and counteracting the devaluation of women that prevails in the sexist, heterosexist, ethnocentric mainstream of psychotherapy and society.

We cannot redefine and transform our lives without changing the context of the culture in which we live. We are coming to a deeper understanding of the ways in which each facet of life, cultural, biological, personal, and political are all enmeshed. To change one is to initiate change in all. The changes women are experiencing today are changing therapy!

Complex Triangles:
Uncovering Sexist Bias
in Relationship Counseling

Joan Hamerman Robbins

*That's quite true, you don't see. You have an absolute talent
for not seeing. Whenever I'm concerned, you don't see, you
see nothing. You look through me, you smile above my head,
you speak to one side of me. And I act as though I didn't see
that you don't see. How clever that is! And how worthy of you
and me.*

Colette, *The Vagabond*

Working with both partners in relationship counseling provides me
with a continuous opportunity to appreciate the profound influence
of cultural conditioning and sex role expectations on people in relationships. As a feminist therapist I thought I had become free of
stereotyped expectations of women and men in relationships. I was
surprised to discover that my behavior in working with couples is
often influenced by cultural conditioning.

In the initial phase of couple therapy I noticed that I was placing
more value and emphasis on male participation than female participation; that I was more concerned with helping a man feel comfortable than helping both partners feel comfortable. I was directing
extra energy at engaging the male partner in an alliance. My
behavior suggested that I accepted the male partner as the person
who held the power in the relationship, and the power to keep the

The author, co-editor of this book, is a feminist therapist in San Francisco where she
works with women, men and couples.

A portion of this paper titled *When Men Talk,* first appeared in The Association for
Humanistic Psychology Newsletter, February 1981.

couple in therapy. These perceptions concerned me and I began to monitor the work more closely.

THE IMBALANCE

In my experience women come to couple therapy with less difficulty and discomfort than men. Many have already been in individual therapy and are familiar with the process of discovering feelings. Frequently they are eager to be in couple therapy and view the counseling as a way to handle the confusion they are experiencing in the relationship.

In general, men are less eager to be in therapy than women. Men have difficulty and discomfort in expressing emotions in the beginning phase of the work. They have been profoundly conditioned by our culture to feel uneasy about expressing feelings and exposing vulnerabilities. They have been trained to be strong and competent, to handle whatever comes up without seeking help. In coming for relationship counseling men are subtly acknowledging that they cannot handle everything; often, in fact they do not know just what is wrong. Men feel sensitive about this and tend to conceal these feelings from others.

I have learned that in this beginning period men will respond more openly to counseling if I remain aware of their discomfort, but do not make it explicit. Masculine "styles" of self-expression have alerted me to the fact that men need a different kind of attention.

> Jeffrey called to ask to come in with Karen, his partner, who is my client. They had talked this over and agreed they would like to see me together. I do not know Jeffrey. I offered an appointment for the following week. Jeffrey responded, "Sure, if we can make it."
> I asked, "Are you serious?"
> He replied, "No, I am joking."

Jeffrey's response tells me that it is his style to use humor to deflect feelings. It could be hard for him to acknowledge that he might feel uneasy coming to counseling with Karen. I will be listening carefully, proceeding slowly, and not making connections too quickly.

As I worked with this imbalance in the early phase of the work, I began to notice a further subtlety. By paying more attention to what men said, I was giving women an equally subtle message: you are less important. I realized that I have been profoundly conditioned as a child to pay attention when a man talked. My father was not very verbal; my mother was the more articulate person in our family. Nevertheless, when my father talked, everyone listened and usually did what he demanded with no "back talk." My conditioning is very deep: when a man talks I pay attention and assume that what he says will be important.

Now I realize the corollary implied: when women talk it is all right to only half listen; they are just rambling and not making much sense. It takes so long for a woman to get to the point.

Part of my skill as a clinician lies in the continuous development of my awareness—an awareness that has evolved through my growth as a woman in our culture, and my identification with the women's movement. These feminist sensitivities blend with my professional training; both are expressed in my paying careful attention to what is happening in the therapy hour, being there for the other person, creating an environment that is safe and comfortable for the exposure of one's self and accepting the other person exactly as she/he is in the moment.

As a woman I have been trained by our culture to do similar tasks. It is often assumed that I will listen sensitively and not speak up; that I will notice other people's feelings and take care of them. In short, it is assumed that I will defer my needs.

In the couples work I came face to face with a dilemma: my conditioning as a woman and my training as psychotherapist were colliding with my deep commitment to feminist principles. As a feminist I am committed to appreciating and acknowledging every woman, aware that stereotyped roles and expectations have often kept us from realizing our potential. I recognized that as I was creating an environment in which a man could comfortably learn about expressing and understanding his feelings, I was inadvertently limiting the woman's arena for self-expression.

What was happening in the first phase of the couples work was reinforcing an old stereotype. We women have been trained to be caretakers; we are conditioned to defer our needs in order to help men express theirs. Most women feel good when they enable a man to express his feelings. We refrain from expressing our thoughts and feelings in the presence of men. We are accustomed to staying silent and waiting to be heard after men have spoken.

The expansion of my awareness of how our conditioning subtly informs female and male roles enabled me to work at correcting the imbalance. Each woman, like each man, requires the same quality of attention to her thoughts, feelings, and vulnerabilities.

Madeline and Tom came into my office ready to begin talking. Madeline hears an inflection in my voice which she interprets as, "You're not ready for us; you're burdened." Madeline says this out loud, enabling me to reconnect to my own feelings. I had just arrived at my office after spending a few days in the country; that first hour back to work is not easy for me. I chose to share this with them, aware that I would be acknowledging Madeline's perceptiveness. Madeline smiles at me, feeling validated. We both bask in the warmth of that exchange.

After a few moments I turn to Tom and ask, "How do you experience this quality in Madeline?" Tom responds, "I marvel at it. I'm really jealous of her sensitivity. I don't know if I can do it; I would like to try and learn to be so sensitive." He is quiet for a minute and then continues, "This obviously would take time and is not a skill I am rewarded for at work."

LESBIAN COUPLES

Same sex couples expand our perceptions about couple arrangements. Perhaps the absence of gender difference provides another view of the issues all couples deal with. The patterns of behavior seem to appear more clearly because the context is changed. Our shared expectations for traditional female-male responses has been suspended.

Some lesbian couples, like some heterosexual couples, struggle with themes of individuation and relatedness: how to handle the pressures and dilemmas created by career, family, and the relationship.

Margo and Alice have been together as a couple for two years. Margo was formerly married and has four children; Alice is a post-doctoral fellow in endocrinology; she often has to stay late at the lab as well as come in on weekends to supervise her research. Margo is a kindergarten teacher and has been at the same school for many years. Her job is routine, comfortable, and familiar. She wants more time at home with her children and Alice.

This couple came to counseling seeking help to deal with the conflicts generated by their different commitments to work. In an early session they hurled pointed barbs at one another. Margo was furious at feeling "like a wife again," always nagging Alice about coming home late and neglecting to help with the chores. Alice was furious with the pressure she felt from Margo and shouted, "I didn't get my PhD to stay home and clean house."

As we explored their different commitments and the feelings elicited by this expression, I noticed a difference from my work with heterosexual couples. What felt different was this pair's commitment to working out their conflicts. With heterosexual couples this commitment generally does not surface as quickly and as clearly.

It is possible that the bonds between women in a lesbian relationship are stronger than the bonds between other partners. Our homophobic culture contributes to strengthening this attachment; people who feel alienated from the dominant culture can draw closer together and provide one another with the support that can be absent from society.

Margo and Alice respected their bond to one another and were determined to keep that in view as they grappled with their upset and angry feelings about the differences between them. *They were creating their own unique model for coexistence in a competitive, hierarchical culture.* Together we were learning about alternatives.

RIVALRY BETWEEN WOMEN

Attitudes and values learned through our early cultural training as females enter the couple work in surprising forms when the therapist is female and the couple heterosexual. It has been important for me to stay aware of the depth and power of this conditioning. If my attention slackened, I noticed that the female partner frequently alerted me to the importance of these themes and their subtle influence on counseling partners in a relationship.

Rivalry between women is convenient for men. We females are so well trained to feel competitive with one another for masculine regard that we do not notice how much attention males require in the presence of females. This rivalry limits our capacity to confront male dominance and assert our own interests.

Rivalry between women for a man is a very ancient part of our female conditioning. Patriarchal culture places high value on a woman living with a man in an intimate relationship, preferably marriage. A woman's successful adaptation to her role is frequently measured by whether or not she has a man of her own.

Most girls grow up fully internalizing the idea that they will marry. Traditionally, in adolescence girls begin to compete with one another for the affection and attention of boys. We accept this competition because the more esteemed goal is to have a male partner. Because of our training women often turn away from knowing one another better; we have been taught to place more value on male attention and affection than female attention and affection. We are deeply invested in this aspect of our female conditioning: attracting, holding, and attaching ourself to a man.

>   The Scotts and I had to change their appointment time because Bill was taking a class that conflicted with our regular hour. Harriet called to ask for an alternative time. When I offered another time she said she would discuss this with Bill and then confirm it with me. Harriet did all this within a short time.
>
>   When the Scotts walked into my office, I began the hour by complimenting Harriet on her efficiency and telling her that I appreciated her efforts.
>
>   Bill interrupted, saying, "I probably didn't appreciate the work that Harriet did." He turned to her, "Thank you." Then talking to both of us continued, "I can do the phoning, but I don't like to do it, and Harriet does."
>
>   Harriet agreed, "I do like to do the phoning for appointments; then I know it gets done."
>
>   I mentioned that in my work with other couples, I had learned that occasionally men have some feelings about making phone calls about arrangements. Bill jumped right in, "It's not that I can't do this, I can do it; but it does seem easier for Harriet since she is at home and she knows our schedules so well." Bill then went on to tell a rambling tale that demonstrated how shy he had been as a boy when faced with a new experience.
>
>   When Bill finished, I turned to Harriet, "What are you feel-

ing now?'' Harriet replied, ''He always does this with other women.''

I sensed that Harriet was feeling very competitive with me and I asked her about that. She acknowledged that she was feeling competitive, and now became aware of feeling jealous of the attention I was giving Bill. She went on: ''This happens a lot in our social life. Bill is always finding women to talk to and tell stories to, and I'm afraid that they will give him something I can't give him.''

Later I realized that when I complimented Harriet, Bill became uncomfortable with the attention she was receiving. He focused attention back on himself and I cooperated. This incident highlights an aspect of female conditioning: *we have been trained to believe that men must always be the focus of our attention if we are going to be the recipients of their affection and acceptance.* It is more comfortable and familiar for me to follow in these ancient tracks than to make new strides.

RIVALRY WITH WORK

Rivalry has many forms. In addition to feeling competitive with other women for male attention, some women feel competitive with a man's work. Work represents yet another barrier to being close to a man. When a woman is not fully expressing her potential in whatever she does, she can overinvest her energy and feelings in her partner (or child). She then expects her partner to fill all her needs and can become envious when her partner finds fulfillment and excitement without her.

Women and men can both be envious and competitive of each other's work. However, it is expected that a woman will ''handle'' the demands and pressures a man's work can place on the relationship. Men do not have quite the same frame of reference when the roles are reversed.

Additionally, we have been profoundly conditioned—first as children and later as wives—that a man's work is very important. He must not be interrupted at work; our ''business,'' whatever it is, can wait until the man is finished with the ''important'' business he pursues in the world outside the home. We are accustomed to being second.

I had first known Sharon several years ago in individual counseling. Now her marriage was in trouble and she was asking for couple counseling; I agreed to see her and Harry. I should have been aware that we would have difficulties because it was unusually hard to agree on our first appointment time.

Sharon arrived promptly. Harry was thirty minutes late. We waited for him to arrive, when he did Sharon blasted him for being late. She was furious. "Why can't you make time for me? Your business comes before everything else and I am fed up with it!"

Harry kept trying to calm her down and make peace with her. He told her that what he was doing would benefit both of them. He took the stance that if only she would be patient it would all work out.

In our brief first meeting, I suggested that Harry might be experiencing some awkwardness. We had not met before, Sharon and I knew one another well; and here we all were sitting in the middle of their troubles. Harry denied that there was anything awkward about this. Yet I observed to myself that the time we had together felt very uncomfortable.

In the first counseling session not being able to help a male client identify the discomfort he may be feeling can contribute to a man being more defensive and his partner becoming more annoyed. Our first meeting will then reflect the impasse the couple is experiencing.

I realized after they left my office that sometimes when men become evasive and deny their feelings I get angry with them and lose touch with my ability to be a sensitive reflector of what is happening in the couple interview. I too grow testy and annoyed; like Sharon I wanted to push at Harry to pay attention.

A few days later Harry and I had to clarify the appointment time over the telephone. I decided to talk this over with him, citing my own awareness and limitations. This led to a very revealing conversation. Harry denied feeling awkward or defensive about being new to the therapy experience or sensitive to Sharon's blasting him. What was making him defensive and angry had been a remark I made about his being thirty minutes late. By my remark I too had shown that I did not understand what goes on for him in a busy day. It was not that simple to clear his schedule and get out of his office; there are countless pressures and Harry did not feel free to just walk out and say, "see you later." He said, "I feel at the mercy of forces over which I have no control."

Harry and Sharon illustrate the heavy price sex-role expectations extract from relationships. In order to survive in the divisions created by sex roles each partner has to deny the value and importance of the other's needs and interests. Harry is handling all the external pressures; he is working hard in order to become successful. With such intense involvement and concentration he is unable to put his relationship in any perspective. He expects Sharon to be patient, loving, and understanding while he is totally engrossed in his business and unavailable to her. Sharon is not able to function under those conditions; she voices the emotional loss to the relationship. *Each partner evidences the limitations created by these roles by feeling out of control and unable to change anything.*

The final vignette illustrates the rapid change in the status of women. Here we see that we do not yet have a framework from which to respond to all these changes.

Helen was talking about her work. Recently she had been appointed to a highly responsible position in her field. She was pleased and enthusiastic about this and went on in some detail. I was listening and enjoying with her her success and competency.

Suddenly, George, her partner, who is also a physician as well as twelve years Helen's senior, got up and said, "I would like to make a phone call; can I use the phone?"

I quickly responded, "No." I went on to suggest that George was feeling left out. "No," George said, "I just heard it all yesterday." I inadvertently interrupted an exploration of how a man feels listening to his partner's success. Instead, I helped George focus on how the issues Helen and I had been talking about related to him. George did not need much prompting, he was ready to talk and be included in the conversation. He began complaining about work: how bored he was with his practice, how he had not felt challenged for some time, and so on.

Later mulling this over, I realized how skillfully we all had avoided dealing with what it does feel like for a man to sit back and *listen* to a woman be proud, successful, and competent. No doubt Helen shared my conditioning; she gracefully backed off and began to listen to George complain. She even asked questions to demonstrate her interest in *his* issues with work. We both slipped back into old familiar roles.

CONCLUSIONS

In a patriarchal culture it has been the custom for men to dominate and women to comply. Not only have we been conditioned to pay attention when men talk, but we have also been profoundly trained not to compete with men. We have learned to relinquish our claims when a man asserts his needs. Women have had more practice in keeping quiet, backing off or retreating than in standing ground 'and demanding to be heard.

This training is deep and complex. Expecting and encouraging a man to dominate is a familiar and safe stance for a woman. We are afraid to challenge male dominance, especially if the male is our partner in an intimate relationship, because we have been taught that challenges to male authority can cost us the relationship.

We have our own inner fears to handle. To demand equal attention can be frightening. Do we deserve this much attention? What if we make a mistake? Will men love us if we are competitive, smart, assertive?

Only now am I realizing how complex it is for women to be role models for one another in the presence of a man. It defies all our training which says that men know better, and even if they do not, we should remain quiet! Until I recognized the influence of my conditioning on my behavior, it was difficult to present an alternative model to other women or to help another woman become her own alternative model.

As I have been working on these themes my awareness has changed and deepened. I now take seriously the profound impact of cultural conditioning on all of us: women and men, clients and therapists. I must continually monitor my own process in order to uncover these biases and change them. It is both obvious and yet subtle. The process demands a willingness to keep in touch with our past, the training received in childhood, and the present interaction. A feminist perspective brings to psychotherapy an expansion of issues and the possibilities for change.

BIBLIOGRAPHY

Gillespie, D. Who has the power? the marital struggle. *Journal of Marriage and the Family,* August 1971, *Vol. 33,* No. 3, 445-458.

Gingras-Baker, S. Sex-role stereotyping and marriage counseling. *Journal of Marriage and Family Counseling,* October 1976, *Vol. 2,* 355-366.

Hare-Mustin, R. A feminist approach to family therapy. *Family Process,* 1978, *Vol. 17,* No. 2, 181-194.

Laws, J. L. A feminist review of marital adjustment literature: the rape of the Locke. *Journal of Marriage and the Family,* August 1971, *Vol. 33,* No. 3, 483-516.

Rawlings, E., & Carter, D. *Psychotherapy for Women: Treatment Toward Equality.* Springfield: Charles C. Thomas, 1977.

Rice, D., & Rice, J. Non-sexist marital therapy. *Journal of Marriage and Family Counseling,* January 1977, Vol. 3, 3-10.

Roman, M., Charles E., & Karasu, T. The value system of psychotherapists and changing mores. *Psychotherapy: Theory, Research, and Practice,* Winter, 1978, *Vol. 15,* No. 4, 409-415.

Tanner, D. *The Lesbian Couple.* Lexington: Lexington Books, 1978.

Wagenvoord, J., & Barley, P. *Men: A Book for Women.* New York: Avon, 1978.

Williams, E. F. *Notes of a Feminist Therapist.* New York: Dell, 1976.

Accumulated Inequalities:
Problems in Long-Term Marriages

Rachel Josefowitz Siegel

Many women and some couples come to therapy as they experience the combined effects of personal transition, family changes, and a rapidly changing social climate. It is a period of transition in which the particular combination of changes is unique for each individual and each couple. Individual coping patterns and couple interactions are severely tested.

My own marriage is thirty-eight years old, and I am still very much in touch with the turbulence and unhappiness we experienced around the twenty-fifth year. It was a challenging and stressful period that led to significant changes for both of us and for our relationship.

The couple who married in the 1950s typically entered matrimony with clearly defined marital roles. He was to achieve and provide, be strong and make decisions. She was to nurture and support, be soft and adaptable. He was brought up to be rational and competitive. She was brought up to be emotional and considerate. If they played it right and worked hard as a team, they might achieve the kind of success that would bring economic security, comfort, and social status. They might be able to offer their children some of the advantages which their parents, coming through the Depression and the war, had not been able to provide.

Mothering and volunteering were a woman's career. Three or four children were not unusual. Child study groups, PTAs, and Cub Scouts were taken very seriously and so was entertaining to further his career. There was no doubt about whose career was primary.

The author is a feminist therapist in Ithaca, NY. She is co-editor of this book, and on the editorial board of *Women & Therapy*.

An earlier version was published in the first issue of *Women & Therapy,* Spring 1982 as "The Long-Term Marriage: Implications for Therapy."

The rare woman who continued to work had a hard time justifying such a choice unless it was out of economic necessity.

Sexually, he was expected to have played around and have some experience; her experience was surreptitious and supposed to be confined to the man she expected to marry. The very topics of masturbation and homosexuality were taboo. The pill was in experimental stages, the IUD not yet available, abortions expensive, dangerous, and illegal. Couples did not live together when unmarried and premarital sexual activity frequently led to pregnancy and a quick and early marriage.

Twenty-five years later this couple is struggling through the mid-life experience in a radically different world. Marital roles are undefined and changing; economic success has brought some status and comfort but not security. The teamwork has cost each partner a high price: their personal development has been one-sided. He has missed the joys of parenting and the relaxation of home-centered activities. She has missed social and intellectual stimulation and opportunities for career development. The kind of mothering she did is now seen as overprotective and self-serving. His involvement with his own career is seen as equally self-serving and sexist. Traditional expectations of heterosexual monogamy are no longer unquestioned. Sexual liberation and experimentation are now acceptable and seen as valuable.

Each partner may well feel a great deal of ambivalence about these changes in the social, economic, and biological environment and about her or his own acceptance of such changes. They may both be very tempted, very anxious, and very unsure about their own and their partner's reaction to change.

Each partner also feels some ambivalence, perhaps anxiety and depression about the personal losses and changes incurred or expected at midlife, and the possibilities of positive as well as negative change involving challenges and unfamiliar risks. As children leave home, they face the prospect of increased intimacy, greater freedom and leisure, a blessing for which they may be quite unprepared. Their personal ambivalence is frequently projected onto the marriage partner who then gets blamed for making changes difficult. The old marriage contract no longer works and renegotiation is complicated.

There are no role models, no signposts to lead the way. Books abound on divorce and widowhood, on single parenting, and on sexual experimentation with both sexes, solo or in groups. It is nearly impossible to find a book on how to maintain and renegotiate a long-term relationship on equal terms. Couples live longer, and if they are still married after twenty-five years, they may feel isolated, unsure, or out of place. Staying married at midlife appears to be very dull; it is nothing to brag about, almost an embarrassment.

The individuals involved in this twenty-five-year-old marriage have now reached a transitional stage in their development and a new awareness of their mortality. The possibility of sudden death or death of a partner becomes a reality and an organizing factor in experiencing and planning for the rest of life even when it is not conscious. This reality may stimulate a wish for more closeness and intimacy or for more distance and separateness in one or both partners.

As we look into some of the losses and opportunities of midlife, it is important that we begin to note the different positions of each partner, for although both husband and wife have experienced some frustrations and disappointments and are experiencing the stresses of midlife, the cards are stacked against the wife. He views the changes of mid- and later life from a position of power and accomplishment, she views them from a perspective of dependency, inexperience, and powerlessness.

The "Matthew effect" (Kirk & Rosenblatt, 1980) explains the accumulation of advantages for men in our society and the obverse accumulation of disadvantages that keep women from ever catching up: "unto everyone that hath shall be given, and he shall have abundance, but from him that hath not shall be taken even that which he hath." I would like to look at the twenty-five-year-old marriage in the light of the Matthew effect, uncovering some of the accumulated advantages and disadvantages accrued by husband and wife, and the ways in which these affect their relationship and their sense of self.

The wife suffers by now from an accumulation of disadvantages that causes severe limitations on the options she has for the rest of her life. Her earning capability is almost certainly much lower than her husband's, she has not had the same educational or vocational opportunities, and her career, if any, has been secondary and interrupted by family needs. If she is widowed or divorced, her situation is economically and socially much more precarious. The interpersonal skills and adaptability which she has developed as a wife, mother, and community volunteer are neither valued by society nor of assistance in finding a job or keeping one; nor do they even provide self-esteem. Her experience in meeting the needs of others, adapting to the schedules of others, and accepting the moves and limitations imposed by her husband's work have not taught her to make her own decisions, to control her own space or time, or to validate or even recognize her own needs and wishes.

The loss of youth which affects both partners may cause him to seek younger sexual partners. For her such a choice is less acceptable and she competes with younger women. She is also at a distinct disadvantage in the job market where a subtle but powerful combination of sex and age discrimination work against her (Sommers, 1974).

The separation from adult children, experienced by both parents with a mixture of sadness and relief, also means the end of a primary role for the mother. The children were her job and frequently also her companions when her husband was away or occupied. The task of redefining herself outside the parental role can be exciting, challenging and very frightening.

She is quite unprepared for the choices and freedom now seemingly available to her. Whether she enters the work force at this point or continues at an existing job, it is at a lower level, with lower status, challenge, and pay than her husband's and with less security for her old age. Her husband, on the other hand, faced perhaps with some dissatisfactions, boredom, or insecurity in his primary role of breadwinner, is not expected to carve out a whole new career for himself. If he does make changes at work, he does so from a position of achievement and the accumulated credentials of a well-established career. He is at the peak of his earning capacity. His situation, if widowed or divorced, is financially much more secure.

Both partners begin to notice physical signs of aging, such as impaired vision or hearing or dental problems, and may have more serious medical problems, such as arthritis, diabetes, heart attacks, a hysterectomy, or prostate difficulties. These health problems, difficult indeed for the patient, also affect the spouse. The worry and fear are there for both, as well as the financial strain, but the wife feels the additional burden of being expected to provide primary care and be nurturing and available in a way that is not expected of her husband. No one would expect him to quit work to make her recovery more pleasant or more comfortable. Similarly, the physical and emotional care of elderly parents falls more directly on a daughter or even a daughter-in-law than on a son. No one expects him to do bedpan duty except under the most extreme circumstances.

Other examples of accumulated disadvantage abound. I would like to consider, as a therapist, the fact that sexist assumptions and role expectations are so ingrained in each of us that neither the wife, the husband, nor the therapist fully realize nor acknowledge the full extent of this marital imbalance, and all three feel threatened at the prospect of uncovering it. The conspiracy to deny these differences, and thus maintain the inequalities, goes hand in hand with a conspiracy to see the wife as the patient and to protect the husband from discovering or exposing his vulnerability, his limitations, and his fear of impotence. We all need to hold onto the myth of a strong male figure, and we also need to deny such a need, for it would uncover our own vulnerability, limitations, and fear of powerlessness.

The polarization of male and female sex roles in our society teaches men to deny feelings of weakness, vulnerability, or doubt and teaches women to focus on such feelings and empathize with the feelings of others. The wife becomes the patient. She feels and expresses the pain, the doubt, the confusion, and the fear that exist for both individuals in the marriage and for the marriage as a unit. She protects us from feeling his pain and confusion. She becomes the patient, the victim, and as such gets the blame.

It is easier to blame the victim than it is to identify the weakness in the system. Both partners collaborate, sometimes with the help of the therapist, in blaming or trying to cure the wife's passivity, neurosis, masochism, lack of assertiveness, and overdependence. I am not advocating that we blame the husband instead, as the wife is frequently tempted to do, but that we examine the differences in upbringing, in opportunity, and in circumstances which entrap both partners in this heavily unbalanced game. In the words of Jean Baker Miller (1976), ''Women become the 'carriers' for society of certain aspects of the total human experience—those aspects that remain unsolved.'' I suggest that as therapists we become aware of the ways in which we add to the accumulated inequalities when we participate in keeping women in this role of carrier or identified patient, and of the ways in which we reinforce the rules of the game and thereby avoid seeing or feeling the unsolved problems of our human experience. We need to be more in touch with our own tendency to admire ''male'' strength and to reject ''female'' weakness because this tendency keeps us from integrating the full range of human experience.

Let me illustrate some of these points with the case of Mary and Tom, who came to therapy after twenty-five years of marriage, aged 46 and 45, with four children ranging from 18 to 24, the youngest just graduating from high school. They had seen a sex counselor who referred them for relationship therapy.

Mary reported a recent hysterectomy, which had become necessary after a severe infection. She was prone to high blood pressure, suffered hot flashes, and was reluctantly controlling these with estrogens. Mary was hurt and angry about Tom's extramarital escapades and his denial of them.

Tom saw no problem in the marriage if only Mary would get off his back, stop rejecting him, stop bringing extraneous matters (his infidelity) into all their arguments. He saw the marriage as far from ideal but would settle for that—why couldn't she? He felt that Mary was overinvested in him and the kids and needed something meaningful to do, perhaps get a job. He came to therapy only under threat of divorce.

Tom was not aware of any feelings about his own midlife transition, nor was he aware of any anger, disappointment, pain, or fear. He did report a dead-end situation at work, having gone as far as he could; he also talked about his father's downhill journey after losing his job at age 45. He saw himself as a rational person and a liberated, nonsexist male, wishing to live the lifestyle of the '80s with an open marriage. He saw Mary as the destroyer of the family, holding her responsible for damaging their four "magnificent kids" with her threats of separation and divorce.

Tom appeared quite sure of himself and of his right to personal freedom within the relationship. Mary was quite unsure of her own perceptions, frequently seeing herself as Tom did, wondering if she was overreacting out of her own insecurity and lack of direction.

After some trust had been established, Mary revealed reluctantly that Tom's escapades began when the size of his erections was no longer as spectacular as usual, though still quite adequate. He had apparently taken some pride in his youthful erectile abilities, which began to wane some three years previously. He began to seek other partners, bringing home a severe infection which Mary believed to be the eventual cause of her hysterectomy. Her present fear of sex and her need to know of his sexual activities were in fact directly related to her fear of being reinfected.

Mary became the identified patient, experiencing both physical and emotional symptoms. Mary and Tom were both troubled by the emotional impact of physiologically determined midlife changes affecting their sexual functioning, changes in family composition, anxieties related to the possibility of new job opportunities, the prospect of other sexual partners, and the fear and temptation of divorce. They were both faced with the existential reality of their own aging, imperfection, and mortality in a society that admires youth and perfection and attempts to deny death.

Tom was able to deny all of these concerns even to himself. Mary expressed them for both. She felt the double burden of carrying the pain and ambivalence of both partners, while coping with the inequalities and disadvantages of her female condition. Mary had become the carrier for the unsolved aspects of their lives and of our society.

During the brief period of our work together, a significant shift occurred in the marital partners' perceptions of each other and of themselves, although the underlying existential problems continued far from resolved.

Mary's feelings and perceptions could no longer be dismissed or invalidated. The effect of Tom's sexual activities on the marital relationship could no longer be ignored. Mary recognized that she would experience severe financial limitations and insecurity even if she found full-time employment before leaving Tom, and that she needed to develop some financial independence if she was to consider divorce as an option. Tom recognized that Mary could leave him, and that he needed to put some effort into the relationship if he wanted the marriage to continue. Mary and Tom no longer automatically assumed that Mary alone was responsible for making the marriage work, nor that Mary was the one who must change and adapt.

As a feminist therapist I found myself in a difficult dilemma in working with Tom and Mary. Was I substituting one kind of sexism for another? Having myself assimilated the cultural messages of our society, I had to cope with my own feelings of doubt and uncertainty, my own female hesitations. Was I invalidating Tom's perceptions when I reinforced and validated Mary's view of the interaction, and when I rejected the pretense of marital equality and the wife-blaming attitudes that Tom and Mary had absorbed from our society? Was I strengthening Mary's position at Tom's expense? I experienced, as Mary did, the fear and self-blame which society has taught every woman, and which transforms an act of female individuation or assertion into the false image of a castrating bitch and destroyer of families. I was breaking the taboo against uncovering male vulnerability. I wondered if it is even possible for a feminist therapist to work with heterosexual couples, when the process of exposing the accumulated inequalities, the existing male centeredness and male dominance may be perceived as favoring the female partner or as imposing female-centered values. When I work with lesbian couples, the culturally indoctrinated and reinforced imbalance does not exist; I break no taboos when I expose the couple's interactive patterns, role conflicts, and power struggles. My own accumulated female rage and powerlessness can be expressed without being misinterpreted as an attack on the dominant or male partner.

When I work with a heterosexual couple I find it especially important to identify my own value system repeatedly, which includes the belief that the growth of one partner, far from diminishing the other, is likely to promote growth in both of them. I also find it necessary to give both partners reassurance, and to indicate that the sometimes painful process of confronting and demystifying their stereotypical role expectations serves the purpose of uncovering and developing previously unknown strengths and important aspects of their individual personalities.

The complicated process of uncovering sexist patterns in relationships and in therapy is an essential element of autonomous nonsexist therapy and requires a constant awareness and examination of the therapist's own attitudes. It also requires an integration of new awareness into the therapeutic interaction, since we have no existing models for nonsexist therapy or for equal marriages.

The case of Mary and Tom illustrates some of the existential realities as well as the accumulated inequalities of long-term marriages. It confronts us with the challenge of helping them find new answers, new patterns of relating in a changing society. In therapy, as in their lives, the rules are changing and we are groping in uncharted territory.

REFERENCES

Kirk, S. A., and Rosenblatt, A. Women's contributions to social work journals. *Social Work*, 1980, 25, 3.

Miller, J. B. *Toward a new psychology of women.* Boston: Beacon, 1976.

Sommers, T. The compounding impact of age on sex, another dimension of the double standard. *Civil Rights Digest,* Fall 1974.

The Role of Politics in Feminist Counseling

Sue Kirk

When we began the Radical Feminist Counseling Component of the Center for Women's Studies and Services (CWSS, one of the nation's oldest and largest women's centers), our concern was not with whether a feminist and radical political philosophy could or should be part of counseling and therapy, but rather with how to integrate a political perspective with the goals and processes of therapy. Thus, one of our major goals was to develop new counseling techniques and to adapt or modify existing ones which were compatible with the tenets and philosophy of the women's movement and the other liberation movements of the 1960s.

To this end we have worked with two kinds of processes for group counseling: the *Creative Solutions Rap Group* (CSRG) and the *Intrinsic, Structural, and Subjective Group* (ISS). Both incorporate the political values of radical feminism in a therapeutic group setting. This article explains both processes.

First, let me describe what we at CWSS mean by radical feminism. Feminism, briefly, is a concern for women's rights and equality, occasionally accompanied by some actions directed towards reform in these areas. Radical feminism, on the other hand, is action-oriented and predicated on an analysis, not only of the plight of women in society, but of the generally oppressive nature of patriarchy, the corporate capitalist system, and the political and social institutions which they have created. It is also predicated on an understanding of how these systems oppress women in particular as well as other groups.

Where the feminist counselor or therapist would ask, "How does the fact of being a woman in a male-dominated society affect the

The author is the Director of the Radical Feminist Counseling Component of the Center for Women's Studies and Services in San Diego, California, and former President of the National Feminist Therapist Association.

psychological and intellectual functioning of the individual?'', the radical feminist counselor would also inquire, "How does living in a patriarchal society dominated by the values and interests of corporate capitalism affect the psychological and intellectual functioning of the individual?''

As we see it, feminist and radical feminist counseling and therapy must not ignore the reciprocal effects of an individual's feelings and behavior, and the social and political milieu. This means that the individual is held accountable and responsible for those aspects of her or his life—and only those aspects—which have a rational or realistic basis for such accountability. A political approach integrated with a therapeutic process does not ignore the uniqueness of each individual and her/his existential responsibility.

For example, it is one thing to maintain, as apologists for the status quo often do, that the woman who is battered or raped usually gets what she deserves, and quite another to have her own up (if there is a basis for it) that she may have acted in ways which made her a more likely target of male aggression—while concentrating on the fact that she is not personally responsible for the violent behavior of her attacker. In cases like this, it is both enlightening and therapeutic to discuss the social, political, and cultural circumstances that so often make women take responsibility for the wrong things, not for the right ones! Thus, radical feminist counseling is not aimed at "laying a political trip" on the person seeking help; rather, at enhancing the dignity and self-determination of the individual.

Furthermore, our counseling processes, including the two outlined in this paper, are meant to provide women with the experience and tools with which to comprehend the political as well as the personal dimensions of existence—and the connections between the two—so that women gain the possibility of transcending, redefining, and transforming their own lives as well as the world in which they live.

THE CREATIVE SOLUTIONS RAP GROUP

In the first session of the Creative Solutions Rap Group (CSRG) the facilitator explains the purposes of the group and outlines the group process. She explains the technicalities, including her role in the group; this involves a blackboard and note-taking. The facilitator then summarizes the ideas and feelings that were expressed during the process. Another participant volunteers to take notes which summarize the content of the session and which will be given to the woman who is bringing her problem before the group. Usually, participants have questions at this point and might want to discuss some aspect of what the facilitator has presented.

At the end of this initial discussion, the facilitator asks each participant to identify some concern, problem, or situation she wants the group to address through the process. If there is still time remaining (each group session lasts for two hours), a participant will volunteer to "go" with her concern. In each meeting there is time for one to two group members to take their concerns through the process. The group will continue to meet until all members have had a chance to share the problem or situation each identified at the beginning, or a new, urgent problem.

At the beginning of the process the woman who is "going" with her predicament shares the particulars of her concern. The facilitator helps her clarify and *focus* the problem. Sometimes, other participants also help with clarification. Although so far this is similar to many initial one-to-one counseling sessions, after the situation or problem has been satisfactorily delineated, the facilitator initiates a round-robin discussion by asking each participant to give feedback to the woman, consisting of *similar experiences and feelings* and how they dealt with them. The facilitator may also participate in this part. Tentative ideas for possible solutions are thus brought out very early and receive further attention later on in the session.

Next, the facilitator asks the woman to identify those aspects of her problem which she feels are unique to her as a woman; or, to put it another way, those aspects of the problem which would not exist if she were a man. Then there is a discussion during which the group endeavors to identify those features of the problem that are common to many women. The facilitator may also share her thoughts and observations on this topic during the general discussion.

Following this discussion, the facilitator asks the woman to try to place the problem in a feminist perspective by "brainstorming" what her life might be like if the conditions and circumstances which contributed to her problem did not exist. What kind of world would she choose? If such a world existed now, how would her life be different?

After the woman has finished developing a vision of her life based on her values, needs, and aspirations (inevitably a world free from the constraints imposed by oppressive and exploitative social, political, economic, and personal relationships and systems), the facilitator initiates a group discussion of the radical feminist perspective. All members participate in this discussion by identifying those features of the problem which are connected to or influenced by the social, political, and economic institutions in which we live. The role of the church, the educational system, the family, the capitalist system, and so on, are examined as they relate to the woman's situation.

After the discussion is over, the facilitator re-focuses the group on the personal nature of the problem in the light of the preceding analysis. The facilitator restates the problem as it was first articulated, and then asks the woman what she feels or thinks about her concern now. In the course of the process, the nature of the problem becomes so much more clearly delineated that the ensuing discussion of creative solutions applies to its most relevant and essential aspects.

Certain aspects of the original concern get resolved during the course of the group process. But sometimes, the nature of the concern changes dramatically, and in the course of re-focusing, the woman may redefine major features of her concern. In any event, the discussion, feedback, and sharing of ideas and feelings have provided the woman with helpful personal insights and new political frameworks within which to view herself and her world. Thus, new options are discovered and possibilities created which open the door to a self-determined, realistic, constructive, and active problem-solving orientation for the individual woman and the group as a whole. Very often, many of the group members have similar or identical problems, predicaments, and concerns. The process which provides the opportunity for one member to explore her concern in-depth also allows others to participate for the time being, vicariously in the examination and resolution of their own dilemmas.

The last part of the process, the "creative solutions" component, is designed to explore the concrete steps the woman may choose to take to ameliorate, if not resolve, her predicament. The facilitator begins this section by asking the woman to state the possible solutions she can identify which involve immediate, intermediate, or long-range change. A round robin discussion follows in which each member is asked to contribute her ideas on what the woman might do to alter her situation. During this section the facilitator reintroduces some of the ideas shared in the earlier feedback from the group, and contributes ideas of her own. The facilitators make sure that suggestions or ideas generated are acceptable choices by directly asking the woman if a particular course of action is feasible for her. In addition, the immediate and long range *consequences* of each possible choice are carefully considered. At the end of the group session the woman is asked to evaluate her experience in the group. The group continues to offer support and serve as a resource to the woman by "following up" on her concern at subsequent sessions.

THE INTRINSIC, STRUCTURAL, AND SUBJECTIVE GROUP

After having participated in a Creative Solutions Rap Group, a woman may decide she wants to continue with counseling by joining an Intrinsic, Structural, and Subjective (ISS) group.

The ISS is a long-term group process for an in-depth analysis of major areas of existence. This group enables a woman to explore herself through writing, in relationship to the social, economic, family, and self dimensions of her life.

1. *The Social Dimension:* This part of the process consists of exploring past and present relationships with other women, men, or children. A woman may use this part of the process to write about the nature of her relationships with specific individuals, sexuality, intimacy, "connectedness," "involvements" with others, social activities, and so on.

2. *The Economic Dimension:* This area includes an exploration of work and work relationships and tasks, employment status, economic dependency or independence, consumer and provider status, and so on.

3. *The Family:* When a group member writes on the family, she deals with her present family, including specific individuals in her immediate family, the immediate family as a whole, relatives and so on. She also examines her past experiences in the family, from childhood to the present.

4. *The Self:* In exploring her attitudes toward the self, the woman answers such questions as: Who am I, sister, mother, lover, friend, etc.? Who am I in relation to men, other women, older people, younger people, people with similar socioeconomic backgrounds,

people whose status is "lower" or "higher," and other people of other races and ethnic backgrounds? What is my relationship to myself? What do I like about myself? What do I dislike about myself? What general patterns of behavior do I perceive in myself? What is my relationship to change?

In most cases, the individual starts by exploring the social dimension, proceeds to the economic, then writes about her family, and finishes with the self.

How the ISS Process Works

The group member writes down a list of relevant specific items she wishes to examine in the area she is working with at the time. If she is starting with the social area, for example, she forms a list of her involvements in social activities and relationships. Next, she ranks each item on the list according to how she feels about the item. If she feels highly positive, she assigns the item a star and places it at the top of her list. If she feels generally positive, she gives it a plus sign and places it under the starred items. If she feels neutral she assigns the item an "o" and places it somewhere in the middle of her list. If she feels negatively she assigns a minus and ranks the item towards the bottom.

Since it is important to account for ambivalence in a person's feelings, the participant is encouraged, when appropriate, to rank items in more than one way. For example, "mother" could be ranked both with a star and with a minus and written about within both rankings.

The woman begins writing about the items ranked with a minus, and she writes about each item in terms of three perspectives: the intrinsic, the structural, and the subjective.

A list in the social area might resemble the following:

* Lisa
* Children
* Joyce
+ Dance Club
+ Bob
o Parties
o Friends at work
o Men
o John

- Friends at work
- Children
- Bruce
- Minnie
- Men

While a list in the family area might look like this:

* Mother
* Aunt Sue
* Brother-David
* Son-Mike
* Daughter-Linda
* Husband
* Father
+ Grandfather
o Mother-in-law
o Cousin-Bill
- Sister-Chris
- Father
- Grandmother
- Son-Mike
- Husband
- Father-in-law

Intrinsic, Structural, and Subjective Dimensions

Intrinsic: When the woman writes about the intrinsic dimension, she emphasizes the *objective* aspects of her concern. She may ask, for example, how social and economic institutions relate to the specific situation or person she is describing in each area. The intrinsic aspects usually cannot be easily changed, except in the long run.

Structural: Next, the group member looks at the structural aspects. This involves an objective analysis of how specific systems, institutions, and circumstances have directly affected the situation or relationship she is writing about. Structural changes are usually easier to make and involve more immediate or intermediate strategies for change.

Subjective: The woman completes her writing on the specific items by describing her feelings about her role in the problem or situation, including her perceptions of that role. Changes in feelings may involve immediate, intermediate, and long-range change. (For examples of writing in each of the three areas, see Appendix.)

After she has finished writing up one or more of the items on her list, the group member shares it with the other members of the group, who, in turn, give her feedback. She may ask the group to give her their responses to certain aspects of her writing. As in the CSRG, the group serves as a source of ideas and emotional support, as well as a possible setting for social and political action and the development of closer personal relationships.

If a group member has a concern which is immediate and is not being addressed through the writing process, she can bring it up at the beginning of the group session. The facilitator of this group primarily assists individual members with writing problems, facilitates the process as a whole, the group discussion, and general feedback. If the need arises, she also meets with individual members for one-to-one counseling.

Both the CSRG and the ISS group provide structures and processes which are dialectical in nature. That is, they begin with the particulars of the individual's experience, move out to an exploration of how the particulars are connected to the larger picture, and return to a focus on the particulars which inevitably have undergone some kind of transformation or modification (e.g., integration of the personal with the political).

Analogously, a member of either group starts by describing her concern in subjective and personal terms, moves on to see how the subjective and personal aspects are linked to the objective or political ones, and returns to take a look at, or experience an integration between the two.

Both group processes develop and maintain a balance of movement between the individual and the group. Such a balance and integration set the stage for action-oriented, problem-solving strategies. This action-oriented approach is backed up, and made possible, by concrete support where the group serves as both a practical resource and a setting for personal change and collective action. It is not unusual for group members to work with each other, or with other organizations, towards changes in the socio-political structures which are, in varying degrees, at the root of many so-called personal problems. A member may start a rape crisis center, begin a childcare cooperative in her neighborhood, work for the passage of the ERA, or run for office.

It would be redundant to stress the consciousness-raising function of groups like the CSRG and ISS. These groups offer a process whereby individual women develop a sense of sisterhood with other women, and a real basis in direct experience for feminist collective consciousness. The process reveals the unity of personal and political motives in an active involvement in efforts to change at least those social, political, and economic structures which are oppressive to women as individuals as well as a group.

APPENDIX

Extracts From an ISS Writing on an Item in the Social Dimension

My Relation to Men (-)

Intrinsic

In this, and most other societies, women are defined by men, for men. Women are "The Other," usually a wife, mother, lover, whore, or child of a man; an appendage to the male for his use or abuse. Patriarchal attitudes dictate social and economic codes whereby men's needs are considered to be primary. *He* is the provider, *he* is the initiator, *he* is the thinker and creator. Women, by nature of their "inadequate" (i.e., inferior) biological makeup, cannot operate within the same realms as equals.

Men control the resources in a world where emotions (women's domain) don't count. Women need to bargain to receive the essentials; women are always put in the role of compromiser.

Men, having the resources and identity to survive perfectly well outside (or in spite of) the relationship, do not have the same kind of feelings of desperation nor abandonment characteristic of the women they relate to.

Women resort to subtlety, "intuition," manipulation, and strategizing to gain some leverage in these relationships. However, women rarely work together or even communicate with each other, because women are seen as competition and are threatening to each other.

Structural

During my first three years in high school, I developed some friendships with some guys. We were a gang of six; four girls and two guys who just bummed around listening to Carole King's *Tapestry* album, going camping and getting sentimental about how neat it was that we were friends. Nick and Robert took turns falling in love with each of us four young women, eventually creating competitive tensions between all of us that severely strained our friendships.

In my junior year in high school, I made up for all the years of non-interaction with men. I developed strangling crushes on a soccer player and on a teacher's assistant named Gary. He was 31, attractive, and he knew it. Our class went camping often, and Gary and I met alone a few times to go sailing. We'd always get very loaded and talk.

The last time I went out with him, he gave me a long line about young women's sexual fantasies and how they (i.e., me) rarely have a chance to act them out. He began to tell me explicitly about his sexual interactions with women and men, and then casually mentioned he was married to a woman eight months pregnant, but they didn't believe in monogamy and wouldn't I like to have sex with a real man, etc. Scared to death with this seduction scene, I quit seeing him.

As a senior, I met Mike, a Texan, who was the first guy to send me flowers and love notes. He was older, handsome, "worldly" (i.e., already out of high school), and he treated me with a "gentleman's respect" (i.e., opened doors for me, lighted my cigarettes, etc.). With Mike, I began to learn more about my body without guilt or fear of pressure to go all the way. I learned to trust Mike, until the day he suddenly left for Texas without notice. Three months later, I got a letter from him saying he'd gotten married to his old girlfriend, whom he'd been engaged to all along.

On the rebound, I went out with Bob, a quiet, serious, intellectual person. But I developed a head cold that didn't go away—gradually he got the message that I didn't want to be "his girl." I again became cold, bitchy, remote: he was a nice guy and I didn't have a logical reason for not wanting to date him.

Subjective

Almost all of my relationships with men have been unsatisfactory. I've hated the roles I've had to play—hated the expectations I felt were *always* there (spoken and unspoken). I never felt comfortable being who I was, because that wasn't good enough. I wasn't the epitome of physical beauty, I wasn't sexually free or experienced, I wasn't unconditionally supportive, I wasn't "feminine" or charming.

I hid behind my intellectual wit. When in doubt, make a joke. Put him down, make a joke. Defend myself, make a joke. My wit was caustic—it gave me a lever, a measure of control, and I *always* felt out of control in my relationships with men. Men had power, they had resources that I needed or wanted. And I envied and resented men for that power.

Each relationship had something to offer me; the guys had something I wanted or admired, and I felt like I was using these guys for my own ends. I'd feel so guilty, ruthless, and scheming. I became convinced that the only way to resolve conflicts would be to have the nice guys quit liking me.

I would try to get them to dislike me by being cold, bitchy, selfish, and irritable. I'd always assume that to tell the guys point blank that I didn't think they were God's gift to womankind, would crush them. Because I did care for them as human beings, and I didn't want to hurt them, I put myself on the chopping block— hating myself and resenting the guys.

Later

There is a part of me which wants to scream "I hate men—I hate them all!" I censor this feeling, this rush of rage.

I feel guilty for being angry and distrustful of men. I feel like I'm supposed to be open. But I'm really scared to be open, it's always ended up shitty for me. And part of me simply doesn't give a damn.

I do know there is a part of me which is curious about having sex with men, but at this point, I'm more confused about the terms of relating with them than anything else.

I don't want to hurt them, but I don't want them to hurt *me* anymore, either.

Women in Interracial Relationships

Janette Faulkner

I had been in Washington one day, walking down Maryland Avenue Northeast with John, when a car full of young black men drove slowly toward us. Suddenly the men made sucking sounds and hand gestures and yelled out versions of "Hey bitch, what you doing with that white boy?" and "Hey bitch, you better leave him alone."

Farther down the street a teenaged black boy bicycled past us, a disbelieving look on his face. "You ought to be ashamed of yourself," he finally said.

To complete the day, that evening a well-dressed black man in Georgetown waited until John took my hand as we left the restaurant before deciding to yell out a phone number to me, adding, "You can call me whenever you need me, baby."

These are some of the humiliations a black woman faces in Washington if her—shall we say special friend?—is white. That's only part of the anguish faced by the increasing number of interracial couples, particularly black/white couples, and most of all couples where the woman is the black partner. The world seems determined to make you feel threatened, angry, defensive, ashamed, lonely, even freakish" (M. McQueen, 1981).

Interracial relationships came out of the closet in the late 1950s. For a variety of historical and social reasons the period promoted an open awareness and sanctioning of interracial relationships between male and female. This very old practice in race relations was not a new phenomenon. The somewhat supportive aspects of society made it safer for some individuals to renew, reveal or experiment with other individuals of a different race, at an interpersonal level.

The author is Assistant Clinical Professor at the University of California, San Francisco Langley Porter Neuropsychiatric Institute, and a mediation counselor with the Family Court Services in Oakland, California.

191

As a Black clinician, practicing psychotherapy in an outpatient mental health clinic, I was particularly aware of the changes. I had the experience of working with women in interracial relationships who needed support and direction around the racism they were encountering because of mate selection. I organized support and self-caring groups and worked intermittently with women in interracial relationships for several years.

In 1975, I observed an increase in the numbers of women seeking psychotherapy concerning issues that could be dealt with in a less clinical, but supportive, setting. Many of these women did not have ongoing support systems where they could verbalize and explore some of their concerns about racial differences. Recognizing this need, I developed a plan with my employer, the Wright Institute (School of Clinical/Social Psychology, and Y-House, the University YWCA) to co-sponsor a series of support groups for the women. The agreement was that the Wright Institute would provide my services as a co-leader. The Y-House, located adjacent to the campus of UC Berkeley, was a meeting place for many women of different racial and ethnic identities, and provided a comfortable, accessible, nonclinical setting for the groups' meetings.

The first group began in September 1975. This paper will provide a descriptive account of the activities, experiences and concerns of the members of seven support groups and the leadership role we provided for a three-year period.

MEMBERSHIP

The purpose of the group was to provide a context in which women could help each other to work with the issues, problems and advantages they experience living with partners and/or children of a different or mixed race, and to train women to co-lead future groups. The group was planned to represent a combination of group therapy (work for individual gain) and group work (work for collective effort or group gain). The early co-leadership was assumed by me and one graduate student from the Wright Institute. We met the leadership requirements of being female, of a different race, with a current or past involvement in an interpersonal (not general, i.e., work, friendship, etc.) interracial relationship. In my past experiences women frequently expressed discomfort around supportive services offered by women who have not shared similar experience. These requirements for co-leadership were a reflection of our sensibility of the newness of the experience and possible inhibitions on the part of the members initially.

The members were recruited via the media and word of mouth. The initial membership requirement was that the members be mothers. We later changed this requirement to meet the request of non-mothers desiring admission to the groups. In the three-year history of the group, screening procedures were not used. This worked very well. In the course of the group experience, there were two instances when we felt a woman needed individual psychotherapy. This observation, plus the recommendation that they continue in the group, was shared by me with each of the women in separate meetings apart from the group.

The groups' size was limited to ten members, meeting two hours a week for ten weeks. At the end of ten weeks, members could renew their group commitment, and at the end of the second ten-week period receive leadership training. One major requirement for this training was regular attendance and active participation in the group experience for twenty or more weeks. A total of 38 women participated in a series of seven separate groups during the three-year period. The attendance patterns were regular and productive.

The racial profile of the group members was 25 White, 12 Black, and one Chinese. All of the black members were married to white males and 24 of the white women were or had been married to black males. The white member married to a white male had three adopted racially-mixed children. The Chinese member had been married to a white male. There were nine single members (all white and never married), five divorced members (four white and one Chinese), and 24 married members (12 white and 12 black). Seven members did not have any children (six married and single white, and one married black). All of the children were racially mixed, representing black/white and Asian/white. The median age of the mothers was 33 years and the children five years.

LEADERSHIP

The leadership requirements, role and approaches to group interaction were based on my clinical sensitivity resulting from past work with other women in interracial relationships and my personal experiences. I have a white godmother with whom I lived and experienced many of the familial and societal concerns expressed by the group members. The first two graduate students to co-lead a group with me were white. One was divorced from a Chicano man and had two children by this man. The other was Jewish, married to an Italian man, and did not have any children. The third graduate student to co-lead a group was black, living with a white man and his son from a previous marriage to a white woman. She co-led with a white former group member. The remaining three groups were co-led by two former group members (black and white) and one former group member (white) with me.

GROUP PROCESS

The initial group encounters by members were very intellectual and somewhat educational, as they shared some of the life experiences of their children and/or mates. We supported this process by encouraging group sharing, asking questions and gradually becoming more self-disclosing about our personal life experiences as related to interracial relationships. We maintained a definite personal responsibility focus rather than a blaming focus that eventually provided a frame of reference for the group members to model. The members gradually became more comfortable talking about themselves, and as a result were less defensive about the sharing process. This supportive atmosphere promoted a mutual sharing by members of some of the sensitive issues resulting from direct experiences of racism. The major themes of the issues were self-identification in a racially different environment, childrearing practices, and societal/familial rejection and indifference toward mate selection. For many of the members this opportunity to share personal feelings and experiences was a "first." It was an opportunity to share observations, questions and concerns with other women with similar experiences. As one white woman stated, "It's a chance to share and support each other around thoughts and feelings that would be viewed as racist in any other setting."

It was important in our role as co-leaders to set limits and rules to facilitate the process and provide and maintain a safe, non-judgemental setting for the group. Some definite limits were set for directive interactions and verbal manipulation exhibited by some of the group members. An example of this was seen in the behavior of the white members who tended to focus on the black members as they shared their concerns about racism and/or their mates. The black members readily accepted the caretaking role and attempted to problem-solve by giving direct advice. We identified this behavior with the black members focusing on their quick assumption of a role white society frequently assigns to them, and a role that they normally would resent. We explained this role as part of the projected image of most women as earth mothers with one goal in life—taking care of their own. For the black women this role projection often carries a double responsibility—that of a super-soulful earth mother who takes care of her own and "white folks too." We followed a similar procedure with the white women, pointing out the negative overtones of their behavior and exploring the possibility that the two groups were recreating some of their societal stress within the group.

We also used this as a time to clarify the issue of control as it often is reflected in the group process. This usually occurs when the large group subdivides into small groups, with one group giving all the power to the other group and yet maintaining the appearance of one group, in that the subdividing is not always overtly observable. We demonstrated this concept by initiating some role-playing exercises so the members could experience the interaction. We divided the members by race into two groups during the role-playing. Each time a white member directed a problem to a black member I would question her choice of focus and my co-leader did the same with the black member who attempted to resolve the problem. Both groups became more self-observing, in that the white members began presenting their concerns and observations as just "that" and not in the form of questions that conveyed a need for an answer, and the black members practiced being less responsive as problem-solvers. The black members tended to ask questions of an exploratory nature, asking how the white member has resolved the problem in the past, and/or they clarified the set of circumstances they were using as the basis of an observation. For example, they used the factual content of the problem as the basis for resolution, and not matter of fact "gut level or earth mother responses."

ARMORING

The armoring process as used herein refers to specific behavioral and cognitive skills used by black and other people of color to promote self-caring during direct encounters with racist experiences and/or racist ideologies. The armoring process is not unique to people of color; however, as a skill it is more developed among people of color because this group is the most stressed by the mark of oppression. I viewed the women in interracial relationships as a group with needs similar to those used by people of color, to deal with their frequent and/or daily encounters with racism. The armoring process as practiced in the group differs somewhat from the approach as defined by persons practicing body work, in that the black and Asian women had been taught and/or acquired the skills in early childhood, whereas the white women were attempting to learn the skills as adults to deal with an element foreign to most of their life experiences—racism.

As a part of the group process, members were encouraged to assume more responsibility for taking care of themselves in the day-to-day negative encounters they experienced in and outside the home. These encounters were usually in the form of a "racist" confrontation questioning the rationale of their mate selection. Many of the white members were often confronted by other whites with, "How did you meet?" "It (the marriage) must have been quite a blow to your parents?" "How could you do this to your race?" The black members were frequently confronted by other blacks with, "Does he have any money?" "Couldn't you find a brother?" "Is that what happens when you go to an all-white school?" Both groups shared experiences of almost total overt rejection of them and their mates, by single, black females. Group members were frequently not invited to social and/or familial activities planned by the women; or not allowed to bring their mates home during the courtship period.

We recognized and agreed with the group that this type of behavior is a common practice among in-laws and friends of couples of the same race; however, these couples experienced the behavior negatively because of the racial differences. For many of the group members the issue of rejection was closely tied in with a loss of network support from family and friends. This was especially true of the white group members, to whom interracial marriage often meant a change of life-style, environment and relationship ties—the latter reflecting a transfer of familial ties to the black families of their spouses. The loss of familial and societal support and/or caring left most of the white members defenseless to an unknown enemy, racism. The white members were taught to take on a new armor, one that protected their physical and emotional well-being from the sting of racism. Historically, western society has provided protection and a "way" for white females to move about and function in a safe environment adapted to the needs and safety of white society. The amount of armor needed for function and mobility in such a socially sanctioned environment is usually very light, and adapted to the general social amenities and interactions with persons of the same race as the wearer.

Western white society does not provide the same protection and "way" for the black female, who in most instances must rely on the family and her immediate external environment for this protection. She is given her armor for racism at an early age as a part of the growing-up process. This acquisition of armor prepares her in a quantitative sense to not only deal with racism, but the issues of loss and rejection because of her interracial marriage.

The armoring process entailed teaching the white members how to be more selective in their use of energy needed to deal with racism; they were taught how to ignore a stare, casual remark or physical gesture, and how to deal with direct verbal encounters and physical gestures. They learned the amount of energy used to respond to direct racial encounters could be determined by the degree of discomfort they experienced. They learned to defend and not exhaust themselves in their frequent bouts with racism.

One white member reported a confrontation with another white woman who spoke limited English. She said, "voo are naught girl. How could you make such zo baby." The member responded, "I can't understand your poor English"—a rather light, but defending, response. However, a similar remark made in clearer English would result in a stronger defensive response such as, "So there will be fewer people like you in this world." Most of the white members prior to experimenting with the techniques of armoring experienced little difficulty defending their children, and almost never had to defend their mates. The newly acquired skills enabled them to take better care of themselves in direct racist encounters.

The black members were taught to exercise more selectivity around the amount of energy used to deal with most racist encounters. They were encouraged to shed and share some of their "armoring" with their spouses and/or children rather than performing the task alone. Some of the black members questioned the probability of a white person being able to "feel and see" racism. One black member expressed repeated disappointments with her white spouse's failure to recognize poor services in public places, a condescending use of first names by service providers, and sexual innuendoes by male co-workers as possible racist gestures. She was encouraged to provide a verbal instant replay of the incident with her spouse each time it occurred, exploring how he experienced it. This type of exploration required less energy, whereas her usual role of dealing directly with the provocateur required more energy and usurped the role of her spouse. This series of exercises was also useful to some white members who expressed concern that their non-white spouses often recognized the racial encounter as such but preferred not to deal with it. In some instances the white members were caught up in the same role as the black members—that of dealing with the incident and usurping the roles of their spouses.

As the group members became more proficient in their selective use of energy, they experienced a productive sense of confidence and mastery over experiences couples of the same race experienced with little incident—for example, shopping, social events, school visits. In general the experience of armoring provided the white members with a sense of feeling less vulnerable outside their homes, and the black members with a sense of feeling less vulnerable in the home setting. This phenomenon may reflect the tendency of both members to remove armor in the home setting and relate to significant others in their usual manner—direct for the white members and non-direct for the black members.

Some white members expressed a feeling of being in complete control in the home setting because "it is *my* setting." White members felt a sense of mastery over the handling of most interactions taking place in the home, including racial barbs from their families or friends or those of their spouse. Some of the black members' experiences were just the opposite. They culturally experienced their home as an expansive environment to accommodate whomever is in it, and therefore would absorb the racial slurs or any other ill-mannered gesture rather than insult their guest, especially if the guest is a relative. Because of this practice there tends to be less of a sense of mastery over friendship, and especially family interactions. In general we interpreted the experiences of mastery as a reflection of different life-style practices between black and white families, in that whites tend to exhibit a more nuclear family focus and blacks a more extended family focus. As an example, one white member had recently asked a distant relative to leave her home because he insisted on teasing her nine-year-old son about his kinky blond hair. A black recalled an incident in her home with her white mother-in-law which left her feeling completely defenseless. The mother-in-law had knitted a set of sweaters and caps for each of her grandchildren. While viewing the knitted items her son noted that a set for his children was not included. He shared this observation with his mother, and her only response was, "Yes, I know." The black member said she was stunned and humiliated by the incident, and was unable to confront her mother-in-law, who remained in their home for several days before leaving to visit her other sons. The incident was not mentioned during the remainder of her stay. Her husband dismissed the incident as one of his mother's eccentricities, adding, "Besides, our kids don't know." The black member experienced the incident as racial, but felt inhibited to respond due to the mother-in-law's age and kinship tie to the family.

IDENTIFICATION

Our racial mixture as co-leaders provided the members with visible models. This racial mixture also provided some support of patterns for maintaining self-identity as a minority individual in the setting of the majority individual. Most of the members upon marriage moved to the host environment of the spouse. This usually meant living in a racially isolated situation. It was a natural expectation that some blending would occur; that is, the taking on of the postural mannerisms, verbal and clothing styles of the majority members by the minority members. Some of the white members were quite at ease adopting a "black style" around body image, dialectical shifting and the use of slang: placing hands on hips, extending and wiggling buttocks as a defensive stance with black and white females. The use of slang and jargon often eased the entry in an unfamiliar racially different social or family setting. The white members using these styles were quite conscious of the shifts and usages, tending to drop the mannerisms when outside of the black community.

The black members tended to assume a more pluralistic approach around self-identification. Their shifts into blendedness were often difficult to recognize, in that most of them came from middle-class families where behavior was modeled after the majority (white) society as a move toward upward mobility. One black member said, "I can be white (affectively) when I want to and black when I want to." Some of the white members tended to identify their children with the race of the father, whereas all but one of the black members tended to identify them as one-half of the racial identity of each parent.

Society tends to identify the child with the race of the non-white parent. One white mother in the group has two children with the same black father. When she delivered the first child she was separated from her husband and entered the hospital alone. The child was listed on the birth certificate as white. At the birth of the second child, she had reconciled with her husband and he shared the birth experience with her. This child was identified as black on the birth certificate. Both children are almost identical in skin color and physical characteristics. A few of the single white members identified their children as black and white with a minimum of emphasis on the ethnic mixtures. One single black member identified her children as "brown." We focused the group activity around establishing a definite identity for the children and reinforcing it with models to support pridefulness. Some storybook and live models were used as sources of identification—for example, Cleo Laine, Van Cliburn, Franco Harris, Viola Wills and Linda Fratianne.

CHILD REARING PRACTICES

The group's major concerns about child rearing practices were definitely racial in terms of parenting roles and parenting responsibilities. The black and white members experienced some conflict with their spouses around discipline patterns. The white members were often criticized for being too permissive with the children and "not making them mind" (obey). Their spouses and in-laws often accused them of creating a false sense of autonomy for the child, recognizing that society does not afford the same freedom and protection for a black child as it does for a white child.

Some of the white members had also experienced similar but less direct criticism from teachers who often referred to the racially-mixed children as being "so physical" (active). Other white members had experienced criticism from older black women in public places, such as: "Girl, why don't you make that boy sit down and be quiet?" or "Those white girls let the kids act like they are white." The black members were often criticized by their spouses for being too strict and by their families for being too permissive. The criticism they experienced from non-related younger and older black women was, "She shouldn't treat those kids like they are white."

The inferences with both sets of experiences are that the white mother is at a loss dealing with differentness and the black mother is trying to take on the differentness.

The group members provided some insightful clarification around the difference between child rearing practices for white parents and black parents. The black members presented the black style of child-rearing based on their own life experiences, as one where the child is taught she/he is "a part of" the society. Interdependency is encouraged as a cooperative effort that promotes individual growth within the society. The goal is to become a vital productive part of the society. The white members shared experiences of being raised with an inference of "being" the society. Independence is stressed by providing a child-centered life-style that supports independence. The goal is to master, control or lead the society. The black child is taught to be obedient and unquestioning. The white child is taught to question and explore; we again see the reflection of the greater society in both patterns of child rearing. The white child is generally afforded the same "way" created for adult whites and the black child is afforded only alternative paths to the "way." The mark of racism blocks any direct paths for the black child to the "way" society creates for the white child.

A general consensus among the black and white members was that while both agreed with these concepts based on their own life experiences, neither was consciously raising their children totally in this manner. The black members felt their current life-style and financial stability was such they could teach and provide a greater sense of autonomy (more than they had received) for their children. The white members felt they were providing more discipline for their children (more than they had received) as an effort to provide them with a means of protection from racism. Role-playing, active problem-solving and mutual advice giving were encouraged to support the members in their child rearing efforts.

The group members expressed some rather generalized concerns about the various stages of childhood—what is a child supposed to be doing at a particular age or level of development. Their concerns were not unlike those of most mothers except they had two additional concerns, race and cultural differences.

Many members needed support and clarification around the question of what is developmental and what is cultural in a child's behavior. One white member was concerned about her daughter, who had a short, kinky, blond afro. The daughter frequently tied dish towels, bath towels, etc., around her head, pretending she had long blonde hair like her mother's. The mother equated this with "wanting to be white" and encouraged the daughter to discontinue this behavior. The mother was relieved to learn from other members in the group that "all little girls with short hair do this, regardless of race."

Another white member expressed similar concern for a teenage daughter who, while in the throes of "Black is Beautiful," rejected her for a black aunt. The members reminded her of their common concerns about race and identity, recognizing that it should not come as a surprise that their children would get some mixed messages about identity.

The group discussed identity issues that all children experience, especially during their teens. The members could readily relate to these experiences from their own childhoods, and shared them. One black member said she had refused to allow her daughter to date black males. In the group she received support around dealing with her own feelings about black males as opposed to exploring possible issues of developmental stages or identification problems.

In conclusion, it is clear that most of the group members were able to explore and role-play some of their expectations about life in a racially different environment. They were supported by the co-leaders and other group members to exercise more risk-taking efforts around dealing directly with racial situations, assuming the parenting role and maintaining focused boundaries around taking care of themselves (armoring). The members were able to establish a support system that has endured and continues to be important in their social and political lives.

Lastly, the goal of training members for group leadership was achieved and the members moved from meeting at Y-House to planned meetings in their homes. The women learned to assume an assertive yet self-caring position around their selection of mate, place in the general society and decisions around child rearing practices. The married and separated women provided models for the non-married women and vice versa, regardless of racial and/or ethnic identity. A network of empathy, rites of passage and creativity was initiated, and continues to provide a support base for members and non-members in the local community, the country and around the world, as evidenced by correspondence requesting information for starting similar groups.

REFERENCE

McQueen, Michel, "The Forces that Tear at Interracial Relationships," *Independent Gazette,* February 1, 1981, p. 2, Berkeley, California.

BIBLIOGRAPHY

Friess, Bernard. "Observation of the therapist factor in inter-ethnic psychotherapy." *Psychotherapy: Theory, Research and Practice,* Spring 1971, Vol. 8, 1, 71-72.

Jacobs, J. H. *Black/white interracial families: Marital process and identity development in young children.* Unpublished doctoral dissertation, Wright Institute, Berkeley, Calif. 1977.

Klein, Judith. "Ethnograph with Jews." *International Journal Mental Health,* 1976, Vol. 3, 2, 26-38.

Kich, George. *Eurasians: Ethnic/racial identity development of biracial Japanese/white adults.* Unpublished doctoral dissertation, Wright Institute, Berkeley, Calif., 1982.

Penderhughes, Charles. *American Journal of Psychiatry,* February 1974, 1312, 171, 175.

Therapists Coping with Sexual Assault

Flora Colao
Miriam Hunt

INTRODUCTION

This paper addresses the counter-transference issues confronting therapists working with victims of sexual assault. The authors are members of New York Women Against Rape, an organization offering hotline and in-person counselling services to sexual assault victims and their loved ones. In addition, Ms. Colao is the founder of the St. Vincent's Hospital Rape Crisis Program, a hospital-based program providing emergency and follow-up medical and counselling services to sexual assault victims. The case histories cited and the observations noted are drawn from working in these two programs.

Given that one out of every three females now alive in the United States will be raped at least once in her lifetime,* and that one out of every four girls in the United States will be sexually abused in some way before she reaches the age of 18 (Weber, E. 1978), the topic of sexual assault is one of great urgency for anyone working with women or children, or both in a therapeutic relationship. It has been our experience that professionals and non-professionals alike fail to recognize the magnitude of the problem.

In recent years, many therapeutic training programs have touched on issues of victimization, particularly victims of violence. However, very little, if any of this information has been from the victim's perspective. This often results in inadequate or damaging treatment for many victims of violence who seek help from therapists. Our own professional training as well as our experiences

---

Flora Colao is the founder of the St. Vincent's Hospital Rape Crisis Program, and is a consultant on the care and treatment of sexual assault victims. Miriam Hunt is a member of New York Women Against Rape, and is currently employed as a psychiatric social worker.

*A mathematical equation based on current population of women in the United States, current life expectancy of 70 years, and FBI statistics on reported vs. non-reported rapes.

as workers in this field have compelled us to raise these issues so that therapists can now begin to recognize and confront them.

A review of the literature reveals that the issue of therapists' counter-transference with clients who have been sexually assaulted has not been addressed. Florence Rush (1980), in *The Best Kept Secret,* identifies the denial by professionals of the importance of sexual assault as a treatment issue, and the high frequency with which it occurs. We cannot overemphasize the importance of this work. In this paper we address the specific issues confronting therapists dealing with the sexual assault of clients.

Definition of Rape

We shall begin by defining rape, both from the legal and the victim's perspective. These perspectives differ radically. Although it varies from state to state, rape is legally defined as forced sexual intercourse, forced on a woman by a man other than her husband* against her will, overcoming her resistance. Definitions of resistance also vary from state to state.

From the victim's perspective, however, rape can be defined as any sexual act performed against the person's will. This would include all forms of sexual assault: anal and oral sodomy, digital penetration, or any form of sexualized physical assault. Clearly, the legal definition does not recognize the difference between compliance and cooperation, nor does it take into account the power dynamics involved in sexual assault.** The kind of help a client receives is inextricably tied to how the problem is defined. Those who would define rape in the narrow legal sense would inevitably fail to notice, much less treat, other clients badly in need of help.

Rape Trauma Syndrome

Most victims of sexual assault suffer from Rape Trauma Syndrome. This is characterized by: intense fear, inability to trust, increased feelings of vulnerability, sexual dysfunction, guilt, shame, rage, increased substance abuse, sleep disturbances (including nightmares), anxiety, suicidal ideation, fear of men and phobic

---

*There are few states in which a man may be charged with raping his wife.

**Legally, only women can be raped. Sexual assault on a male is not considered rape. We deplore this, but for the purposes of clarity—and also because the vast majority of sexual assault victims are female—we will refer to victims as "she."

reactions (Burgess, A., & Holmstrom, L., 1974). Any or all of these symptoms may be manifested. If these symptoms are not recognized and treated, the client may remain in crisis for years. Symptoms of Rape Trauma Syndrome can appear pathological to someone unfamiliar with the syndrome. If the therapist does not recognize the reactive nature of these symptoms, she/he may misdiagnose the client.

It is also of crucial clinical importance that the trauma of sexual assault, even when dealt with therapeutically, can still be reactivated. That is, when a woman is in a situation dynamically similar to the assault (i.e., her autonomy is being threatened), she may manifest the symptoms. On the other hand, she may not manifest these symptoms, but may experience similar feelings of anxiety as she had shortly after the assault. It has been recognized legally (Homes vs. Aryee) that rape results in permanent psychological injury. This issue is just beginning to be recognized in the professional literature; Baum, Shore, and Sales (1982) speculate, ". . . it seems necessary to consider whether a trauma as severe as rape results in permanent psychological damage."

In psychoanalytic training, therapists are taught to view discrete incidents as part of a client's life pattern. Therapists, who like everyone else, have internalized the victim blaming myths of our society, may view rape as part of the personality pattern of the victim. Hence, some therapists will talk to a rape victim about her "self-destructiveness" or her "masochism." In addition, since the frequency of sexual assault is denied by society as a whole, therapists may view the client with suspicion; Did this really happen? Is it a fantasy? Did she provoke it? Did she enjoy it and now feels guilty about that? Why is she "overreacting" to or "obsessing" about the rape? Is she trying to use the rape to divert me from the "real issues"? Is she trying to seduce me with this "sexual" information? Is it a good lesson for her?

D., a 16-year-old rebellious adolescent, was gang raped at 2 a.m. in an area where she had been forbidden to go. She had been in therapy for two years because of her "antisocial" behavior. After the rape, she became the "model girl"; her grades improved, her substance abuse stopped, and she obeyed all her parents rules. Her therapist told her father, "We could never get through to her. The rape is the best thing that could have happened to her, because now she understands what we were trying to protect her from." One year later she was admitted to a hospital emergency room after a suicide attempt. The "model girl" behavior was likely masking feelings of fear and rage after the assault. There could have been more successful intervention had the therapist helped D. separate the issue of her rebelliousness from the issue of the rape.

Crisis Intervention for Victims of Sexual Assault

The crisis intervention counselor deals with the sexual assault as a discrete incident in the woman's life. The emphasis is on returning the client to her previous level of functioning. The counselor in a crisis setting has the responsibility for recognizing serious emotional difficulty and referring the client to a long-term therapist skilled in dealing with these issues. Unfortunately, there has not been enough communication between rape crisis centers and therapists. Consequently, there are still too few therapists trained to effectively deal with rape victims.

The reality of sexual assault is that it is a life-threatening experience. Victims frequently feel that they have faced their own deaths. Rape is a life-changing experience for the vast majority of survivors. The victim needs to mourn the identity she feels she has lost in the assault. This is similar to the grief reaction following the loss of a loved one and must be treated sensitively. For some clients short-term intervention is enough, for others long-term therapy is the answer.

SPECIFIC ISSUES CONFRONTING THE THERAPIST

There are many reasons why therapists are unprepared to deal with these issues. We have already mentioned the dearth of theoretical and practical education offered to professionals. But there are other, more subtle, factors. One of the biggest is the amount of mythology surrounding the issue of sexual assault in this culture. A few of these myths are:

— Rape is a sexual act.
— Women provoke or incite attack.
— Women never get raped by men they know.
— Women invent stories of rape to get men in trouble.
— A woman is not seriously affected by a rape unless she is physically injured.

— Women secretly desire rape. You can't rape a woman unless she really wants it.

These myths have long been disproven by people working in the field of sexual assault. However, professionals, as members of this society, may have internalized these myths and unconsciously perpetuate them in their work with clients.

A related issue is that therapists have not been trained to recognize that blaming the victim is a way of protecting themselves from feelings of vulnerability and their own fears of sexual assault. What commonly occurs is that the therapist begins to project his or her own myths about sexual assault onto the victim. In addition, classic psychoanalytic training has exacerbated this tendency. Few of us in our professional training have been taught to question these myths, much less question what purpose they serve.

Specific Issues Confronting Male and Female Therapists

A female therapist, confronted by the client's assault, may respond with her own feelings of vulnerability and fear. She may remember a sexual assault in her past; she may become angry, whether or not she's conscious of it, at her client for raising these issues. This anger may take several forms. Some therapists, displacing their feelings of vulnerability, become over-protective and controlling of clients, which prevents clients from regaining control of their lives, a necessary step for recuperation. This also prevents resolution of the crisis. Others find themselves restricting their own lives. Some also restrict the lives of other clients or close female loved ones.

A male therapist, confronted by a client who has been assaulted, might feel guilty about being male. Often, the male therapist finds himself needing to prove that he is a good man (unlike the rapist), and seeks reassurance from the client at a time when she needs to concentrate her energies on herself. This can be done very subtly, most commonly by encouraging the woman to recall good experiences with men. He also may offer physical comfort, without realizing that it is his needs that are being met by such behavior. He may feel guilty about his own past sexual aggression, rape fantasies or attraction to his client. Vulnerability is also an issue for the man; he may find himself over-protecting the women in his life as well as his other female clients. It is painful to realize that people one loves can be sexually assaulted and that sexual assault can happen to any woman. All of this may result in anger at the client for raising these issues in the therapist.

Therapists who are unfamiliar with this subject often fail to recognize or know how to cope with their feelings of discomfort. A therapist might realize that she/he is angry at the client or unable to focus with the client on her feelings related to the assault. She/he may feel guilty about that, not understanding that these are normal responses, that there are reasons for them and that they can be dealt with.

Specific Issues for the Client

After a sexual assault, a client is in crisis. She is experiencing at least one, and most likely several of the symptoms of Rape Trauma Syndrome. She wants and needs therapeutic intervention desperately. Simultaneously, she is feeling extremely vulnerable and therefore realizes the precariousness of her position, should her therapist respond inappropriately as by invalidating her feelings. Some clients, sensing their therapist's inability to cope with this crisis, will simply withhold part or all of the information.

R. went into therapy at age 16 after a gang rape. Because she sensed her therapist was uncomfortable with the details of the assault, for three years she did not disclose that her friend had been murdered during the rape.

Many clients fear that the therapist will view the rape as part of their life pattern. Many women have said to us, "I can't tell my therapist because she/he is always telling me how self-destructive I am."

L., a 32-year-old woman had a sexual relationship with a man she had been dating for several months. One night they returned to his hotel room after a date. To L.'s horror, there was another man waiting in the room. Her date left her with the man who raped her repeatedly. L. told her therapist of the incident the next day. His response was, "Why do you suppose you keep getting into these situations?" She had never been raped before and had had no reason to distrust the man she had been dating. If this therapist did indeed believe that this woman was self-destructive, the time to explore that would be after she had been restored to her previous level of functioning. To ask such a question at this point could only intensify her stress.

B., a young actress had been raped. She was worried that because she was attractive, she was somehow "marked" for assault. In attempting to make a referral, we called one therapist who said, "Well, that (her attractiveness) probably has a lot to do with it. She's probably been giving out vibes that attract men."

Clients have also internalized society's myths about sexual assault. Because of this, the client and the therapist may end up colluding in blaming the victim. This burden may be exacerbated by efforts to follow inappropriate advice from the therapist, for example, suggestions that she resume usual behavior patterns before she is ready, or that it is now time to move on to other "more important" therapeutic issues.

Clients have also internalized the myth that the therapist is powerful and omnipotent. When in crisis, this myth is very important to them and can lead to unrealistic expectations about what the therapist can do to solve the crisis. When the client discovers that the therapist cannot take the pain away immediately, the response is often rage. If the therapist is unprepared for this rage or is unattuned to the seriousness of the incident which prompted it, she/he may lose the client without either of them understanding why.

All sexual material is highly charged for the client at this time, particularly if there is confusion in her own mind between sex and sexual assault. If the therapist shares this confusion, the situation is volatile. If the therapist uses previously-divulged sexual information (e.g., masochistic or incestuous fantasies) to explain the assault, or to interpret the client's reaction to it, the client often experiences this as betrayal and violation. Any sexual innuendoes and/or physical overtures, no matter how innocently meant, may also be experienced as abuse by the client.

P., a 27-year-old woman, took a cab home from a party at which she had been drinking. She had decided not to take public transportation as she felt that since she had been drinking, she would be safer in a cab. The cab driver drove her to an unfamiliar area and raped her. After several months she told her therapist about the rape; she had held off because of her own guilty feelings connecting the drinking with the rape. Her therapist asked, "Did you enjoy it? I have to know if that's part of your guilt." This is an example of how therapists have internalized myths about rape, which then become part of their counter-transference.

Another important counter-transference issue for some therapists is the need to feel that the client has overcome the rape experience. This can result in feeling threatened if the client brings up the rape when the therapist feels it should be a closed issue. Some therapists have asked us, "Why is she 'holding onto' the rape?" or will suggest to the client directly, "It's unhealthy to dwell on this." Sometimes a therapist's own feelings about sexual assault can be so unresolved that she/he can either deny the client's experience or the impact it has had.

S., a self-defense instructor, began remembering a frightening incident with sexual overtones from her childhood. She wanted to explore this with her therapist. Her therapist said, "People like yourself, working with rape victims, often want to identify with their students and will fantasize that they have had similar experiences. Just forget it, it probably never happened." She changed therapists. After six months with a therapist who helped her explore this memory, she was able to unblock the full memory of a rape that occurred when she was 8-years-old which had been documented by her childhood medical records.

TRAINING

In our experience, clients' intuitions that their therapists will not respond sensitively to the news of a sexual assault are well-founded. Most women who tell us that they are afraid to bring incidents of sexual assault to the attention of their therapists are afraid for good reason. The case examples are unfortunately all too typical; we assume they reflect ignorance rather than malice.

We encourage therapists to take a training course in rape crisis intervention. If that is not possible, it would be wise to become familiar with the currently available information about rape from the victim's perspective and the psychological effects of sexual assault on victims.

In our experience, conducting courses on rape crisis intervention, we find that therapists frequently exhibit more discomfort than do non-professional students. This may be for several reasons. It is difficult for many established professionals to assume the role of student and to learn about an important issue that has been explored and clarified mainly by non-professional women. More accustomed to the role of providing help, therapists are often uncomfortable asking for help when the material feels overwhelming. This may lead to denial of the intensity of the feelings or even withdrawal from the course.

What seems to be most difficult for professionals to accept is the validity of the political implications of doing effective therapeutic work with victims of sexual abuse. Many therapists do not see their work in a political context and therefore resent it when such connections are made. However, we feel that it is impossible to work with victims of sexual assault without considering the context of women's role in a patriarchal culture. The classic analytic viewpoint simply does not address the severity nor the scope of the problem of sexual assault in this country. Sexual assault is the extreme enactment of "male" and "female" roles as they are learned in this culture.

Males learn that they are expected to be aggressive, powerful and controlling. Females learn that they should be submissive, passive and dependent on males. In a sexual context, men and women learn to view each other's and their own sexuality in a proscribed way. Men learn that they are expected to take what they can get, to view sex as one of many conquests. Women are taught that it is their role to control the expression of their own and male sexuality. Since she is expected to depend on males, the woman is put in the position of having not only to control male sexual aggression, but to depend on males to protect her from it. In the sexual assault situation, the woman is confronted with the brutal reality that she cannot count on male protection.

The challenge for the therapist, especially after a sexual assault, is to re-enable the woman to function independently in a society that discourages independence. Given woman's socialization, her independence, resourcefulness, and survival skills are stunted. Lacking these survival skills and viewing herself as weak, she is at a disadvantage in general in society, but especially in the sexual assault situation. The frequency with which sexual assault occurs would suggest that there will never be an end to it until the damaging polarity between what is considered male and female behavior is eradicated.

CONCLUSION

Sexual assault is occurring at an alarming rate in this society. All therapists undoubtedly have clients that are or will be at some time trying to resolve feelings regarding sexual assault. The victim-blaming myths of our society have been internalized by clients and therapists alike, and affect the therapeutic relationship. Therapists who educate themselves to the victim's perspective of sexual assault and to the counter-transference issues will be more effective in helping clients in the recovery process.

REFERENCES

Baum, M., Shore, B. K., & Sales, E. Rape crisis theory revisited in Weick, A., & Vandiver, S. T. (Eds.). *Women, power, and change.* Washington, D.C.: National Association of Social Workers, 1982.

Burgess, A. W., & Holmstrom, L. L. Rape trauma syndrome. *American Journal of Psychiatry,* 1974, 131:9.

Holmes vs. Aryee. 81 Civ 0777 (RWS). U. S. District Court, Southern District of New York.

Rush, F. *The best kept secret: sexual abuse of children and adolescents.* New York: Prentice Hall, 1980.

Weber, E. Sexual abuse begins at home. *Ms Magazine,* May 1980.

ADDITIONAL READINGS

Bard, M. *The crime victim's book.* New York: Basic Books, 1979.

Burgess, A. W., & Holmstrom, L. L. *Rape: crisis and recovery.* Maryland: Robert J. Brady Co., 1979.

Griffin, S. *Rape: the power of consciousness.* New York: Harper & Row, 1979.

Groth, A. N., *Men who rape.* New York: Plenum Press, 1979.

Horos, C. *Rape.* New York: Dell, 1974.

Medea, A., & Thompson, K. *Against Rape.* New York: Farrar, Strauss, & Giroux, 1974.

Russell, D. *The politics of rape: the victim's perspective.* New York: Stein & Day, 1975.

Sgroi, S. M. et al. *Sexual assault of children and adolescents.* Massachusetts: Lexington Books, D. C. Heath and Co., 1978.

The Reality of Incest

Janet O'Hare
Katy Taylor

New York Women Against Rape (NYWAR) has been counseling victims of sexual assault since 1973. When we first began to receive calls from children who were the victims of incest or from adult survivors, we had little understanding of the problem. We quickly learned that the existing literature was limited and damaging. We also discovered that many of our clients were afraid to tell their therapists about this most fundamental victimization. Some had been told by their therapists that the incest was a fantasy growing out of their unresolved ''Electra complexes''; others that they had enjoyed or provoked it.

We realized that the only way we could learn about incest and how to help its victims was to listen to the survivors themselves. While we were learning from the survivors of incest, other rape crisis centers and feminist oriented helping agencies were also going through a similar growth process. They, too, have been developing methods for identifying and treating victims of incestuous sexual assault. In 1976, with the help of pioneering therapist Robbie Stuart, we began running incest survivor support groups. These groups have taught us the reality of incest.

We define incest as any act with sexual overtones perpetrated by a needed and/or trusted adult, whom a child is unable to refuse because of age, lack of knowledge, or the context of the relationship. Prolonged abuse by a babysitter or an old family friend, even if limited to inappropriate bathing or kissing, may prove as traumatic and may produce the same symptomology as abuse by a blood relative. Either type of abuse may foster feelings of lack of

Janet O'Hare is a member of New York Women Against Rape, and a major organizer of NYWAR's annual conference since 1980. She chairs the Training Standards Committee of N. Y. City Advisory Task Force on Rape. Katy Taylor was the originator of NYWAR's Incest Program. She edited the sixth issue of *Heresies, Women and Violence*, and is now consultant for Working Women's Institute.

control over bodily integrity, fear and incomprehension. Similarly, a sexual assault such as being made to watch one's father masturbate can be as traumatic as being made to have intercourse with him. It is important for us to shed our "copulocentric" view of incest and other kinds of sexual assault.

Incest happens frequently and in all neighborhoods and families, although only a fraction of incest cases come to official notice at the time of the abuse. There are no reliable statistics; if one were to make a biased judgment based on the women who first sought NYWAR's help in resolving their incest experiences, one could conclude, contrary to widely held belief, that children of executives and physicians from wealthy Connecticut suburbs were more at risk than those of ghetto dwellers.

We will refer to the victim of incest as "she" and the offender as "he." Based on our research, however, it is reasonable to assume that prepubescent children of both genders are equally vulnerable to sexual abuse. It has been our experience at NYWAR, that males are more likely to block the memory of childhood abuse from consciousness, while females are more likely to have these memories triggered by sexual assault in adulthood.

The vast majority of offenders appear to be male but there are women who sexually molest their children as well as mothers who cooperate actively or passively with their husband's abuse of their children.

Males who have experienced sexual abuse as children may have the same symptoms associated with female survivors. Some men may replicate the abuse they have suffered on their own children and/or other children who are accessible to them. Some male survivors have worked to explore and end the abuse of children.

In this paper we will discuss the myths about incest which are accepted as true among many therapists, to the detriment of their clients; the reality of incest as it happens; the symptomatology of past and present incestuous abuse and the implications for treatment.

THE MYTHS

Incest is a Child's Fantasy Rather Than an Adult's Behavior

The most important and destructive myth is the Freudian one which deals with incest as a child's fantasy rather than an adult's behavior. Peters (1977) and Rush (1976) have discussed in detail the way in which Freud backed away from his original correct perception that incestuous abuse is often the cause of hysterical symptomology. Possibly as a defense against this unacceptable reality, he developed his theory that all children experience sexual desire for their parents without examining the feelings and behaviors of parents toward their children. Modern and often vulgarized interpretations of Freudian theory have led many therapists and lay people to deny that childhood "seductiveness" is learned and may stem from incestuous abuse.

Incest Only Happens Among Social Outcasts or the Psychologically Disturbed

It is not unusual to hear professionals dismiss incestuous abuse as characteristic of poor communities' "culture." Another theory focuses on the pathology of the individual offender of the family, and attempts to explain incest as a by-product of alcoholism, schizophrenia, or generalized family violence. Incest does occur in families prone to many forms of violence. It also happens in families who are less likely to be referred for treatment.

In our experience, incest perpetrators are often socially esteemed, e.g., doctors and executives, individuals defined as normal by society and their community. If offenders undergo psychological testing, they tend to test normally.

A "Bad Mommy" is Responsible for the Abuse

This theoretical trend, which blames the mother instead of focusing on the offender, has been analyzed in detail by Butler (1978). The literature contains many variations on this theme. Sometimes the mother is accounted "bad" because she didn't know about the incest (a "good" mother is supposed to know everything concerning her child's welfare). The fact that the offender and the victim used every possible means to keep the abuse a secret appears irrelevant.

Sometimes the mother is "bad" because she knew and didn't do anything, even though she lived in life-threatening fear of her violent husband, knew that existing social services were worse than useless, or knew no way of supporting her children without the aid of the abusive husband. These factors are rarely considered in the literature.

Sometimes the mother is "bad" because she is unable to fulfill her proper role and (often "unconsciously") forces her husband to sexually abuse their daughter. The wife's frigidity and sexual rejection of her husband are frequently cited as causes—that the husband may have been a brutal marital rapist is again deemed beside the point. Of course there are elements of these situations in some incestuous families—some mothers are "bad"—but to assume that incest is caused by such behaviors is erroneous and highly destructive.

When appropriate case histories are taken from offenders and victims, it is frequently discovered that the offender himself was abused or exposed to sexual abuse as a child. Offenders frequently begin to abuse other children by early adolescence. As they grow older the age and status of their victims can expand. Sometimes the learned pattern of abuse is being repeated in the homes of at least some of the survivors' siblings children.

We believe that no one commits one isolated sexual assault. The rates at which individuals commit their crimes vary greatly from the man who regularly commits one isolated sexual assault. The rates at which individuals commit their crimes vary greatly from the man who regularly rapes wife, children, female and juvenile male relatives, as well as an imposing number of acquaintances and strangers on a regular basis, to the man who desperately tries to restrain his behavior and only offends under stress. However, it is imperative that judges, therapists and family members recognize that there is absolutely no reason to believe that the offender will cease sexual abuse until he is in therapy *for sexual abuse* conducted by a therapist *expert in this problem* and this has proved effective for the offender.

While the family dynamics may indeed be inappropriate in an incest family this is the *effect* of incest not the cause.

Special Daughter Theory

Much of the literature focuses on a "special daughter" theory. Although many offenders do indeed tell their victims that they are "special," this does not mean that they are not also abusing their other daughters, sons, or even the neighbor's children. Sometimes all the children in the family, male and female alike, are abused in the same way, and sometimes the sons are taught to abuse or sanction the abuse of their sisters. In either case it must be assumed that any child is at high risk when accessible to the offender.

Some Types of Incest are Worse than Others

According to this theory, brother/sister incest is the least destructive type, father/daughter incest not so bad, and mother/son incest the most damaging, particularly when intercourse has taken place.

Our experience indicates that all incest is destructive and individual responses are determined by other things than the exact relationship or the type of acts performed. The idea that brother/sister incest is not harmful comes from confusion between the consensual sex play of prepubescent siblings of similar age and the exploitation of a child by a much more powerful person. Experiences of the former type are common and often seem to produce no ill effects. There is some clinical indication, however, that post-adolescent sibling incest seems more likely to occur in families where there is sexual abuse. Our clinical experience does not indicate that women (or men) abused by older brothers show fewer ill effects than women (and men) abused by their fathers.

Affection Theory

Recently the popular press (*Penthouse,* December 1977 and *Time,* September 1981) has reported a movement supported by some professionals and congruent with notions of free love and sexual liberation espoused by some members of our society, to encourage the acceptance of sexual relations between adults and children. We have no quarrel with adult relatives, freely choosing to be sexual with one another on the basis of mutual noncoercive attraction. However, the idea that a child can ''freely consent'' to be sexual with a parent or another adult is ludicrous.

Proponents of the affection theory argue that the child is at least getting sexual information/education at home and receiving affection. These arguments are popular with offenders and are often invoked when the child tries to resist the abuse, or, if the abuse is disclosed, to justify the abuser's behavior. What the child learns by being used to fulfill an adult's fantasy has no relation to the child's needs and developing sexuality. Its adverse effect is borne out by the large numbers of incest survivors suffering from diverse forms of sexual dysfunction.

The defect in the ''affection theory'' is that the child learns that ''love'' is what an adult wants to take from her, not what he wants to give to her. The child is taught that sex is a tool for manipulation and domination.

Many practitioners are still influenced by myths about incest. It is unusual to find an incest survivor who has not experienced some sort of inappropriate intervention from therapists, particularly those survivors who began the search for help over five years ago. In addition to miseducation, most therapists are unwilling to deal with their own fears and longings about incest; like all of us, they experience strong emotional reactions when faced with the topic. Confronted with horror (and perhaps an inadmissible sense of titillation) at the violation of one of the most important taboos in every culture, and the gross unfairness of sexual abuse of children by those who should be protecting them, the human mind seeks ways to pigeonhole or perhaps discount the unwelcome information. This helps insure the continued vigorous health of many of the damaging myths about incest.

THE REALITY

There is tremendous variation among families that experience incestuous abuse. However, many of the following elements turn up regularly in our case histories at New York Women Against Rape: Incest is virtually always repeated, usually on a regular basis for many years. All sexual offenders recidivate and the notion that the offender's children are his undisputed property encourages him to assert his rights whenever he chooses. It is common for the earliest remembered incest to have started at around ages five to seven (although there are many cases where the overt incest begins in infancy), and to continue on a gradually escalating scale, often coming to include various forms of penetration and frequently coming to some sort of crisis at puberty.

Puberty is a time when boys who reach the offender's size are often able to extricate themselves from the abuse. Girls frequently make an attempt (or an additional attempt) to tell their mother or someone outside the immediate family. Now they are alarmed at the possibility of becoming pregnant themselves, or that the offender will extend his abuses to younger siblings. Sometimes the threat of telling is sufficient to end the incest—at least for that child. Sometimes the family controls are so tight that the oppression will continue through adulthood and into new generations. Sometimes the sexual abuse is part of a total complex of family pathology involving psychosis, drug abuse, and other forms of violence. Sometimes the incest involves severe physical abuse and constant threats of death.

Incestuous families often replicate the classic "model" family, with a clearly defined hierarchy, the husband/father maintaining control over much of his wife's and children's behavior. Often the offender is a pillar of the community and the family is very concerned with keeping up appearances.

In the beginning the child doesn't know what is wrong. There may be a variety of bribes, or simply the pleasure of adult attention. Grown-ups do many strange things, why not this? But the child quickly learns that this must be kept secret. She also learns over time that it is a bad secret; by keeping it she, too, is bad. Some children, of course, are inured to abuse and survive by complying with each order. As they grow older they begin to learn that they have broken a taboo and that they are indeed bad. They learn from their teachers, their doctors, their families, and from the offender that it is best to pretend that the taboo wasn't broken, or not very badly, or that it was not very important.

Child abusers who commit incest have different approaches. Many are brutal but most seem to prefer more subtle forms of coercion. Enlisting the child in some sort of forbidden but desired behavior insures both compliance and guilt. New behaviors are generally introduced gradually as the child is trained to act out the offender's fantasy more fully. This approach provides great opportunities for rationalization, "she loves it, she asks for it," which have fueled the confusion within the therapeutic community, "she was obviously willing—it went on for years—she never told anybody about it."

The offender will tell the child that she is special, that the game is their secret, that the incest is necessary for her health, that he's doing it because he loves her, adroitly playing on the child's desire to be loved and fear of losing affection. The abuse is often a regular event when the mother is absent, or can take place when she's sleeping in the next room (sometimes even in the same bed). As the behavior escalates and as the offender (often) grows bolder, the child may come to realize that she has a certain bargaining power over this adult. (Incest survivors often feel most comfortable with men whom they can manipulate.) Sometimes as the abuse continues the child will start to respond sexually to the stimulation. Offenders perceive this as complete justification for their behavior and the victims perceive their response to the stimulation as betrayal by their own bodies.

Sometimes the child is truly "special" and the other children in the family are not being abused. Often, however, they are being abused unbeknownst to one another. Different siblings may have different reactions to and effects from abuse by the same relative at the same time. The incest isolates siblings from each other as well as from their parents.

However, an attempt to rescue younger siblings from sexual abuse is the most common reason victims report the abuse to outsiders.

When children do attempt to get help the results are often disastrous. Young children lack the language to describe what is happening to them. Children's attempts to communicate are often totally misinterpreted. One child drew a stick figure with an enormous erect phallus and was told by her furious kindergarten teacher never to draw such dreadful pictures again. Another child told her mother that grandpa was always bothering her and her mother replied, "You bother him too."

Children learn to split themselves in two as a way of living with this secret for which they will be (or have been) punished for revealing. They must maintain the facade of normalcy or be held responsible for destroying the family. They often have one self that goes to school and church and Girl Scouts and another self that feels the pain. They may split themselves off from all bad thoughts and feelings and attempt to become perfect. Some children deny all societal rules and become perfectly bad. They may run away often or permanently. They may be recaptured by a pimp, the juvenile court system, or an early marriage and babies.

Our experience with incest has taught us that children may not remember fantasies and may minimize real repercussions from sex with the parent because they have organized massive defense efforts to block awareness of incest from a hostile world. Far from not experiencing anxiety, such children devote tremendous amounts of energy to keep anxiety from showing and to maintain the appearance of normalcy. Current victims and adult survivors have developed defenses of incredible strength in order to survive. The unacceptable knowledge will often be blocked from the conscious mind once the behavior has ended. Between incidents of ongoing abuse this unacceptable knowledge can remain blocked only to resurface later during some life crisis. They may forget the incest entirely or crystallize it into a single event or a much shorter period of abuse. The trauma will remain in place until another crisis shakes it loose, or until a time of great stability and courage enables the survivor to seek out a safe person to tell her story. Current victims and survivors are accessible to intervention anywhere along the way. Walking into any high school classroom and mentioning the existence of rape within the family will almost always reveal a youngster or two who knows all too well what the speaker is talking about.

Decoding the Message: Learning the Signals

In addition to the symptoms already known by professionals to indicate other forms of child abuse there are signs that indicate incest. Since we believe it is vital for all those in the helping professions and all those who work with children to be familiar with these symptoms, we will list a few important ones. They are: in children and adolescents: conversion hysteria, phobias—particularly of men and certain individuals, sleep disturbances, excessive bathing, splitting behaviours, obsessions or phobias regarding sexual matters, public masturbation; in older children: sexual abuse of younger children, seductive behaviour toward adults, chronic urinary tract infections, venereal disease or pregnancy, delay or disruption of menstruation, vaginal, anal or urethral bleeding; in adults: compulsive behaviour, severe difficulties with intimacy and trust, sexual problems—especially difficulty integrating mind, body and feelings, feelings of being a freak, poor body image, amnesia about childhood, guilt and shame, severe contempt for, and hostility and distrust towards men especially of one's own ethnic group, phobias of being touched—gynecological exams, fear of losing control.

The therapist who observes a cluster of such symptoms in a client and thinks that she/he is an appropriate source of help should proceed slowly, with caution, and allow the survivor control at all times. It is unlikely that the whole memory is readily accessible and it may be buried if the therapist shows signs of being overwhelmed or of not taking it seriously. The key is to remain calm, matter-of-fact, and accepting. These things happen to a lot of people; they are painful but they can be dealt with. Incest victims can and do recover.

If the person is trying to unblock the memory, she should be helped along gently. These are some questions to ask: "Do you think you might have ever been physically or sexually abused?'' ''Did it start off fairly mild and get worse?'' ''Was it just you or do you think he was doing it to the other kids too?'' ''Did he give you the feeling that it must be kept a secret?'' ''Have you been able to find anyone to help you with this problem?'' *The key is to listen.*

It is good to offer a survivor the chance to tell the details to a calm professional who is not going to become upset, and will respect the importance of taking the cues from the survivor. There is a tendency for the professional to want to get the ''facts'' about acts committed and not pay enough attention to the much more important facts about how tyranny was maintained in that household. Many therapists are attracted to the use of hypnosis to help clients remember details of the incest. We do not recommend this unless the survivor feels totally in control of the hypnotic trance and is expert in its use. It has been our experience that incest survivors will unblock memories as they need to in a supportive environment. It can be devastating to remember the whole horror at once and patience is appropriate in dealing with a problem that was years in the making. Healing is a long-range process, and it is important for the survivor to be able to continue functioning in her daily world.

All children should be routinely asked: ''Does anyone ever touch you when you don't want them to?'' Affirmative answers must be checked out. When incest is discovered, a careful assessment of the family situation is necessary. There is no hard and fast rule about whether the child or the offender should be removed from the home. Being sent away often feels like punishment to the child—and the child may end up in another situation just as abusive. It is also traumatic to feel responsible for Daddy being taken away by the police. Many incest survivors say that the ''help'' provided their family by the designated agencies ''broke up the family.''

A compassionate approach to the entire family and reassurance that its members are not alone is helpful. The therapist (or a trusted person acting as therapist with the help of a professional) can determine who in the family is most supportive of the child and can offer help to that person. A professional is mandated by law to report child abuse but the legal situation should be carefully explained to the family. The offender should be referred for treatment and it should be made clear that if he seeks treatment it will be included in the report.

Children should not only be protected from further abuse but they should receive a clear explanation of what has happened that is appropriate to their level of understanding. Children need extensive opportunities to "discuss" the incest in words, in drawings, and in play. Efforts should be made to reforge family alliances damaged by the isolation of incest.

TREATMENT

Every therapist with a large practice must assume she/he is treating incest survivors. Many of these clients are afraid to reveal their victimization because of previous bad experiences with therapists (although some simply do not remember). Many survivors have learned that some therapists cannot "hear" about the incest even when it is described in so many words, while others dismiss it as an irrelevancy from the past inappropriate for current discussion. Others are so overwhelmed and horrified that the patient drops the topic out of pity. Of course, many therapists respond with variations of the myths stated earlier. Many persistent survivors, determined to receive help, may try ten or fifteen different therapists until they find one who is able to help them. Often the therapists that help know very little about incest; however, they do know enough to throw away the textbook and listen to the client.

To respond appropriately to incest survivors in a therapeutic situation, the therapist must honestly confront her/his feelings about sexuality (especially child sexuality) and the incest taboo. If the therapist has been psychoanalytically trained, that training can be a tremendous handicap in working with an incest survivor unless it is thoroughly reevaluated.

Control and autonomy are key issues for incest survivors. A controlling therapist is too similar to the incestuous abuser to be helpful. In addition, many survivors, male and female, have difficulty relating to male therapists, and male therapists often have great difficulty relating to incest survivors. Many female therapists can also experience problems in relating to survivors. If a survivor chooses to change to a female therapist this should be seen as a positive sign of taking control and not as inappropriate avoidance behavior.

The goal of therapy with an incest survivor is to help her assume control over her own life. The therapist is there to support the client and help her empower herself. It's very important for the therapist to help the client recognize her own strengths in order to use them to confront what she had previously used them to deny. The therapist must respect the client's own healing process and allow that healing to proceed at the individual's own pace. *The survivor is the ultimate expert on her own condition.*

Incest cannot be understood and treated solely as an example of isolated familial pathology. It must be placed in its social and political context and that means in a feminist context. Like other forms of sexual assault, incest is a crime of power and coercion; one of its cultural functions is to maintain the power structure of our patriarchal society. The relation of incest to other forms of family violence and the oppression of women, children and vulnerable men is not irrelevant to treatment. This means that one cannot effectively cope with the overwhelming guilt and feelings of being a "freak" which incest survivors experience, unless one has a perspective informed by a broad understanding of the actual practice and function of incest in our society.

As the therapy progresses, the therapist must continuously reassess her/his own reactions. What does this bring up from her/his own childhood? How are these feelings going to affect the therapeutic process? The likelihood of the therapist unblocking assaults of her/his own is fairly high while working with a survivor. The more one learns about sexual assault the more one realizes that we are all affected by this problem.

Support Groups for Incest Survivors

We at New York Women Against Rape have found our incest survivor support groups to be of tremendous help, even for those people already in effective individual therapy. Incest survivors are haunted by the difficulty of separating the problems in their lives which are caused by the incest from those which are not. The support group provides an opportunity to sort this out and to heal the shame and isolation that cannot be eased in any other setting. Incest abuse often causes a severe lack of faith in oneself, and the group provides a means to build and confirm that faith over and over again.

However, the groups are not suitable for everyone. The survivor must be ready to give as well as to receive. The survivor, who, at long last has received an appropriate response, wants to get that support again and again. At this time survivors must have the chance to tell their story repeatedly without having to worry about other people. Many recently unblocked survivors go through a period of "verbal diarrhea." Robbie Stuart (1976) says: "For every time you wanted to talk about it and couldn't, you need to talk about it now."

We have found from our experience with incest survivor support groups that when establishing a group it is a good idea to avoid having just one member of a particular subgroup: e.g., Black, lesbian, mother, older person, etc. Isolation within the group is to be avoided as much as possible.

Our group facilitators are selected from highly experienced rape crisis counselors who have proved successful in working with groups. In order to establish the fact that not everyone is a victim of incest and to remind the group that problems can emanate from other sources, we generally have two facilitators: a survivor to provide safety and trust, and a non-survivor to break the secrecy.

The role of the facilitators is to encourage and sometimes direct group interactions. Focus on the facilitators as "experts" is to be avoided. The group members are all experts on their own experiences. The facilitators serve to make sure that the basic ground rules are followed:

1. The establishment of trust and safety for the members is predicated upon confidentiality of group process.
2. Listening respectfully provides the opportunity and encouragement for individuals to speak, therefore, interruptions and judgments are not permitted.
3. To prevent defensiveness and insure feelings of safety, anger is to be directed only at the facilitators and not at other group members. The facilitators make sure that the focus of the group is maintained and that everyone gets a chance to speak.

The facilitators encourage group members to take responsibility for the group and each other; for example, exchanging telephone numbers and suggesting topics for discussion. Since incestuous assault affects all aspect of the survivor's life, the group will deal with a wide variety of topics: trust (of oneself and others), self-image, sexual functioning and relationships. Role playing and discussion of survivor's current problems are important tools practiced in the group.

Powerful feelings emerge in the group. Anger, grief, shame and isolation are exposed in this safe space. All feelings are allowed in the group, including positive feelings toward the offender.

An area that is very difficult for survivors to cope with is the sexual arousal that some victims experienced during the years of abuse. Examination of this aspect of the abuse may shed light on a survivor's sexual problems and may even upset the comforting illusion of mechanical sexual "functioning." This can be overwhelming if the facilitators are not ready to help. *It is vital that the therapist/ facilitator express clear acceptance of the fact that a survivor's physical response to prolonged sexual stimulation as a child was not tantamount to complicity.* The survivor may feel the betrayal by her body as "proof" of such complicity, but in fact, as the therapist/ facilitator must stress, it is a perfectly normal response to the situation.

The group is structured so that each participant can move at her own pace. Facilitators watch for a "backlash response" when a member goes farther than she has previously in talking about the abuse in the safety of the group. The survivor may become terrified at the risk she has taken and become angry at the group or facilitator, or feel the need to retreat.

Every session begins with a few minutes of assessing how everyone is feeling since the last meeting and a discussion of any issues that arose during the week. Each session ends with a quick stocktaking of the group interaction, focusing on the positive and checking to see how everybody is feeling.

CONCLUSION

Societal horror at incest and the mythology perpetuated by experts, have blinded many practitioners to the incest that is all around us. Incest is not a rare deviation, not all of its victims or offenders are psychotic. Therapists see the effects of incest—distrust, depression, sexual dysfunction—in their clients every day and are unable to alleviate these symptoms because they don't know where they come from. Helping incest victims requires us to educate ourselves, clarify our values, and practice those values. It requires effective treatment programs in every community for child victims, secondary victims, adult survivors and offenders (all of both sexes).

It is time that we share information among the helping professions and rid ourselves of our prejudices against practitioners of different backgrounds. It is especially important for credentialed professionals to listen to grassroots rape crisis counselors who often have more experience and knowledge in this area. Expanding community education programs, especially for children and those who work with them, is also crucial. Most of all, it is essential that we talk to our children about sexual assault, and provide them with the information that they have to know in order to control their own bodies. Further, no doctors, teachers, relatives or parents have the right to violate that control. Children must be taught that they have a right to talk about sexual assault.

Incest must be confronted. It is being faced because incest survivors, with the support of the antirape movement in particular, and the feminist movement in general, have had the courage to break the silence, tell their story, challenge misinformation and to share their pain and their strength with their sisters and brothers.

REFERENCES

Butler, S. *The conspiracy of silence—the trauma of incest.* San Francisco: New Glide Publications, 1978.

Leo, J., & Galvin, R. M. Cradle to grave intimacy. *Time,* September 7, 1981, 69.

Nobile, P. Incest. *Penthouse Magazine,* December 1977.

Peters, J. Children who are the victims of sexual assault and the psychology of the offender. *American Journal of Psychotherapy,* 1977, *Vol.* 30, 398-421.

Rush, R. The Freudian coverup. *Chrysalis,* Spring 1976, *Vol.* 1, No. 1, 31-45.

Stuart, R. Personal communication, 1976.

ADDITIONAL READINGS

Abel, G., Becker, J., Mercer, W., & Flanagan, B. "Identifying dangerous child molesters." In R. Stuart, *Violent behavior.* New York: Bruner Mazel, 1981.

Blumenthal, R. Did Freud's isolation, peer rejection prompt key theory reversal? *New York Times.* August 18, August 25, 1981, cl.

Burgess, A. W., Groth, A. N., & McCausland, M. Child sex initiation rings. *American Journal of Orthopsychiatry.* 1981, *Vol.* 51, No. 1, 110-119.

Lesbian Mothers' Custody Fears

Terrie A. Lyons

Lesbians are veiled in myth and misconceptions as the media and popular culture portray them as masculine, narcissistic and psychologically impaired. The lonely, self-deprecating women depicted by many novelists, as well as stories told in hushed tones about "diesel dykes," form the backdrop for the development of many of the stereotyped images of the lesbian today.

The assumptions that these images have in common are: (a) lesbians deny their own femininity, (b) they attempt to emulate men through masculine sex-role behavior, and (c) they hate men. These extreme or stereotyped conceptions of lesbians act on an actual and symbolic level to challenge traditional sex-role expectations, defying what is expected of a "real" woman. Thus, in the extreme, the lesbian represents for all women the refusal to be submissive to men.

If lesbians are seen to contradict what is expected of them as women, then even more do they contradict the behavior expected of them when they are also mothers.

LESBIANS AS MOTHERS

If lesbians cannot get close to men, how can they be mothers? Their children are proof of their histories with men, and their marriages, either present or former, reflect heterosexual courtships and relationships. In what manner can these "unfeminine" women, who are typically seen as hedonistic (or should I say "shedonistic"?) obsessed with sexual gratification, be altruistic, nurturing mothers—the ultimate reflection of femininity?

The author is a Licensed Clinical Social Worker in private practice, and is currently completing her doctoral work at the Wright Institute in Berkeley, California.

The research reported in this paper was carried out under NIMH Grant No. MG 30890.

The author wishes to thank Ellen Lewin for her comments and editorial assistance on the final draft of this paper.

Using Kinsey's estimate, approximately 10 to 11 million American women are lesbians. Other authors (cf., Martin & Lyon, 1972) postulate that about 20-30% of lesbians are also mothers. Thus the total number of lesbian mothers in the United States is approximately 2 million. The proportion can be expected to be higher in large, liberal metropolitan areas. The largest number of lesbian mothers become mothers through marriage. Following a trend in the general population for unmarried women to intentionally bear or adopt children, a growing number of lesbians are having children on their own or with their women partners. This is accomplished through adoption, artificial insemination or various kinds of relationships with men. These relationships with the father range from strictly instrumental sexual encounters to cohabitation or common-law relationships.

THE AUTHOR'S RESEARCH ON LESBIAN MOTHERS

Between 1977 and 1981 my colleague, Ellen Lewin, and I conducted a comparative study of both lesbian and heterosexual mothers, focusing upon the different kinds of support systems that they employ to meet both emotional and material needs for themselves and their children. Relationships with family, ex-husbands, lovers, children, friends, and agencies and institutions were examined to understand both their supportive and conflictual effects on family members. The first phase compares 80 lesbians and heterosexual (43 lesbian and 37 heterosexual) formerly married mothers. One-half of the lesbians and one third of the heterosexuals live with partners.

These mothers have been matched for age of children, relationship status and socioeconomic status. The second group of mothers, for which data analysis is not complete, represent lesbians and heterosexuals who have never married. This paper focuses on the experience of the formerly married mothers.

RESULTS

We found no differences between the lesbian and heterosexual single mothers in the area of social support systems. The lesbian mothers were just as likely as their heterosexual counterparts to call upon their parents, the child's grandparents, for a variety of resources, such as childcare, money in financial emergencies, or lessons for the children. Depending upon geographic proximity, the grandparents were involved in varying degrees with mothers' lives, no differently for the lesbians than for the heterosexuals.

Relationships with ex-husbands also showed few differences. The relationships with the ex-husbands ranged from very friendly and supportive to hostile or non-existent. However, no differences were correlated with sexual orientation.

For those who had co-resident partners, concrete support with childcare, money and household management, as well as ongoing emotional support, was usually provided by that partner, regardless of sex. Thus, male lovers, were just as likely as women lovers to shop, babysit and share the emotional responsibility for their partners and their children; they were also equally apt to generate family disputes or to be jealous of time mothers devoted to their children.

The only major difference we found between the two groups of mothers was the lesbian mothers' concern for loss of custody of their children. Fear of loss of custody was a persistent theme which arose in discussing various aspects of the mothers' lives.

Fear of being "brought out" or exposed as a lesbian in a work situation raised anxiety. Sally, one of several teachers in our sample, taught in a local preschool. Although her employer knew of her lesbianism, she lived in continual fear that a parent of one of her pupils might discover her lesbianism and force her dismissal. The loss of her job would not only create problems in her career, but the lack of income would make her more vulnerable to possible attacks by her ex-husband.

The possible discovery or disapproval by ex-husbands of their affectional preference was a further area of concern for the lesbian mothers. This fear of disclosure and consequent challenge of custody caused many mothers to be circumspect about the details of their lives, both to their children and their ex-husbands.

In examining the data, concern for loss of custody may be categorized according to actual experience of litigation, threat of custody loss and generalized fear of custody disputes. When we consider those women who actually went to court over custody issues, we find that the lesbian and heterosexual mothers are not very different.

However, in threats of custody dispute not involving actual litigation, sexual orientation does make a difference. Sixteen percent of the heterosexual mothers had been threatened with loss of custody, while for the lesbian mothers, 33% had been threatened either by their ex-husbands or by their in-laws with the loss of their children.

In nearly all cases, the mothers' sexual orientation was the reason for the threat. In total, slightly less than half (46%) of the lesbian mothers had either been involved in custody litigation or had been threatened with such action because of their lesbianism.

Although more than half (54%) of the lesbian mothers had never been to court or threatened with litigation, nonetheless, almost all, expressed fear that they could lose custody. For example, one mother who had been separated from her husband for two years, explained the elaborate plans she developed to insure that her lover and husband would not meet. While she had not actually been confronted by him about her life-style, she lived in continual dread that he *might* find out, and be compelled to sue for custody. Thus custody, whether it has been litigated or not, is a central theme in the lives of lesbian mothers. Their concern about custody must be understood, not only in the context of their own lives, but in the broader legal experience of lesbian mothers.

LEGAL ISSUES AND CASES

The legal standards which prevail in child custody actions set them apart from other areas of the law. Each case is judged on its own merits with individual circumstances examined closely. When a lesbian mother wins a case, no precedent is set which would affect the outcome of similar cases. Additionally, custody can be challenged by the ex-husband, grandparents, or any interested party, such as neighbors or governmental agencies who might be concerned about children being raised by an "unfit" or lesbian mother. In these cases, the state can step in and try to determine how fit a mother is and how suitable the home is for the children.

In addition custody awards are never final. The standard of "material change in circumstance" can be raised to review a custody determination at any time. This means that when such factors as the physical setting, the mother's or father's life-style, or their marital status have changed, the previously arrived at custody arrangement may be returned to court for reevaluation. Thus, for lesbian mothers, not only the actual change, but the discovery of their sexual orientation may prompt custody action.

Finally, the legal concept of "the best interests of the child" is the standard by which custody is determined. This standard is determined by the subjective judgment of the judge as to whether or not a particular parent, home, or circumstance enhances the best interests of the child. Most important in their thinking has been the question of whether the child will grow up to be homosexual or without the appropriate sex-role behaviors of a boy or girl in this society. A secondary concern has been that the child might be stigmatized or teased because of his/her mother's homosexuality. Judges have also worried that there might be sexual misconduct in the home of the lesbian mother. Further, because judges are also prey to the stereotyped images of lesbians, they may have doubts about the ability of a lesbian mother to be maternal.

Various legal writers, notably Hitchins (1979), and Rivera (1979) have described lesbian mother custody cases. Rhonda Rivera documents a rise within the last five years in the number of lesbian mother custody cases that come to court. One frequently made stipulation in cases where custody may be awarded to the mother, is that the mother is forbidden to see her lover in the presence of her children. The presumed intent of this condition is to protect the children from the full effects of the mother's homosexuality.

In a California case (Chaffin vs. Frye, 1975) the judge was required to determine the custody of two adolescent girls, ages 16 and 13. Instead of focusing on the mother's criminal record and her social and financial instability, the judge cited her homosexuality as his reason for awarding custody to her parents. In doing so the judge commented "this factor is not merely fortuitous or causal but rather it dominates and forms the basis for the household in which the children would be brought if custody were awarded to her. The mother does not merely say she is a homosexual, she also lives with the woman with whom she has engaged in homosexual conduct and she intends to bring her daughters up in that environment. . ." He also showed concern that the children would be exposed to homosexuality "during their most formative and impressionable years." Aside from the judge's distorted knowledge of child development, the interesting point in this case is that the judge chose to award custody of both daughters to the only adults in the courtroom who had proven that they could raise homosexual children, as both the mother and her brother were homosexual! (Lewin, 1981).

Effects of Custody Cases on Lesbian Mothers

A particularly important effect of these legal decisions is their impact on the consciousness of lesbian mothers. Publicity concerning these cases has often been picked up by the newspapers, and even, in recent years, by television. For example, the Mary Jo Risher case, which was tried in Texas in 1977, was recently portrayed in a major television movie. Although this movie presented the lesbian characters in a positive light, and was in fact, a sympathetic portrayal of their lives, Mary Jo Risher's loss of custody of her son very likely heightened anxiety among lesbian mothers. This dramatic presentation, like news stories, in a similar vein, confirms lesbian mothers' fears that they could never get a fair hearing and that continued custody of their children may be precarious.

Custody as blackmail. One of the concrete effects that this awareness of the legal experience of lesbian mothers has is to make any threat by ex-husbands, either overt or covert, a realistic possibility. Mothers in our study, for example, have agreed to adjust their property settlements in exchange for an understanding that their lesbianism will not be brought up in court. One mother spoke bitterly about losing her house and agreeing not to fight her ex-husband about her fair share of the equity in the property, for the understanding that her sexual orientation would not be raised in court and her custody would not be challenged. In other cases, mothers may give up rights to spousal support or simply not sue ex-husbands for back child support payments. For example, a number of mothers in the study have hundreds and in some cases, thousands of dollars in back child support payments owed to them. They are reluctant to take legal action against their ex-husbands or to attach their wages for fear they will use the lesbianism to gain custody of the children.

For mothers who are very concerned with possible loss of custody, extreme secrecy about their lesbian lifestyle must be maintained. They hide this information from their ex-husbands, and may also worry specifically about reactions of grandparents, school authorities, and even their own children. Further, some mothers worry about their children's awareness of their sexual orientation because the children may reveal it to their fathers and grandparents.

This fear of disclosure can have major disruptive effects on the comfort and ease of family gatherings, the degree of intimacy with the family of origin, and communication between mothers and their children. Family therapists have examined the family rules surrounding a "family secret" and the ways in which the sense of something terribly wrong (but unspoken) in the family can be internalized by the child as his/her own defect (Haley, 1977). Thus, depending upon the degree of secrecy and unconscious guilt surrounding the mother's lesbianism, the child is likely to internalize a sense of shame or "wrongness" without consciously knowing the cause.

Externalization of other fears. The psychological process of introjection and projection may also operate in the lesbian mother. Being oppressed as a woman with a sense of powerlessness in the world, when combined with discrimination against lesbians, such as rejection by her parents or fear of losing employment, may be internalized as a personal feeling of worthlessness or helplessness. This low sense of self-esteem, concerns for providing adequately for her children, and other anxieties and fears may be projected out onto real, documentable events. For the lesbian mother, the custody battle can be just such an event. She has seen and read about it happening to other mothers; it can happen to her. When this fear is combined with possible threats or feared threats from her ex-husband, loss of custody in the mind of a lesbian mother, is not only a possibility, but becomes an event anticipated with great anxiety.

For example, one mother I interviewed told me that her remarried ex-husband, did not spend much time with their children. In addition, his new wife did not even like his children. From all external appearances he would not be likely, at least in my estimation, to return to court to fight for custody. Yet in the mother's mind this was a real probability. As we talked further I began to see that her concern with his challenging her custody was linked to her feeling out of control in the world. After many years she had gone back to school, and had concerns about fully supporting her children. She felt ambivalent about wanting to be more independent and having three young children dependent on her. Moreover, the interview revealed some discomfort with her lesbianism and a preoccupation with being "deviant." These anxieties and fears were projected out by her and expressed in concern for the loss of custody. Thus, for this informant, loss of custody had become both an internalized and an externalized symbol of the consequences of her lesbianism.

Being a mother is the central organizing factor in the identity and lives of both lesbian and heterosexual mothers; being a mother was perceived as being more focal and primary in effecting daily living and concept of self than race, economic factors, living situations or sexual orientation. Furthermore, the birth of their children was cited more frequently than the divorce or coming out as major turning points in their lives. Motherhood is the most significant life event which bonds both groups of lesbian and heterosexual single mothers.

It is this sharing of the common bond of motherhood which sets lesbian mothers apart from all other lesbians and gives them more in common with women with children than similarities in race, economic status or sexual orientation. One lesbian mother put her feelings as follows: "Being a mother to me, being a mother is more consuming than any other way I could possibly imagine identifying myself. I am a lesbian mother, I'm a working mother. The word mother hardly ever modifies anything. Mother is always primary, it is always some kind of mother, but it's never a mother anything." For these mothers of both sexual orientations motherhood was not only the most primary part of their self-identity, but, because of its importance, was also the area in which they felt most vulnerable.

Implications for Treatment and Advocacy

Separate fear from fact. One of the tasks of a clinician working with a lesbian mother who has custody concerns is to help her realistically weigh factual data and distinguish them from her fears. How much time does her ex-husband spend with the children? How interested is he in his children's activities? Does he pay child support? And if so, does he do so reliably? Does his new wife or lover like the children? Does he use the children as a vehicle for power or anger against his ex-wife? How much of her concern is a response to external threats and how much may her anxiety embody other fears?

Along with an appraisal of outside factors, internal concerns must be assessed. How does the mother feel about her ability to provide for the emotional and physical needs of her children and herself? Does she discuss her lesbianism with her children, and how does she deal with any feelings which may arise? What effect does her lesbianism have on other relationships with family, ex-husband, and others? What is the relationship between her lover and children? Her lover and her ex-husband? As in any psychotherapy, the therapist must be sensitive to not only the external pressures on their client, but the internal, emotional consequences of those realities.

Legal consultation. Although only a small percentage of lesbian mothers actually face custody litigation, the clinician may be called upon as a consultant to lawyers in a lesbian mother case. As an expert witness, the clinician may be used to educate the court about sexual and gender role identification, socio-cultural aspects of lesbian mother families, child development theory, and to evaluate family members. The performance of these roles will depend greatly upon how familiar the therapist is with clinical issues in lesbian families and with the most current research concerning lesbian mothers and their children.

CONCLUSION

Lesbians are characteristically seen only in the light of their family of development. Their psychological relationships with their mothers and fathers are examined and analyzed as though only their past exists in relation to family. It is only in the wake of the women's and gay liberation movements, and the notoriety lesbian mother cases have received in the media that lesbians have gained visibility as mothers. Researchers, (Hoeffer, 1981; Kirkpatrick, 1981; Lewin & Lyons, 1982; and Mandel et al., 1979), have just begun to explore the complexity of roles and relationships in the lives of lesbian mothers and their children, contradicting the masculine and developmentally arrested image of the lesbian popular in the past. They have documented more similarities than differences between lesbian and heterosexual single mothers.

In particular, research indicates that motherhood, rather than the pursuit of multiple lovers, is the central organizing theme in the lives of otherwise ordinary women. The struggles of providing housing, childcare, money, maintaining employment and raising their children, unite rather than divide lesbian and heterosexual single mothers. Only in putting aside our preconceptions about them as lesbians, can we appreciate the impact and stress of these structural factors and begin to understand the lesbian mother in the context of her role as woman and mother. It is incumbent upon us as therapists to struggle with our own prejudices and stereotypes about lesbianism and motherhood in order to allow the full complexity of our clients to emerge.

REFERENCES

Haley, J. *Problem solving therapy.* San Francisco: Jossey-Bass, 1977.

Hitchens, D. J., Martin, D., & Morgan, M. An alternative view to child custody: when one parent is a homosexual. 17 *Conciliation Courts Review,* December 27, 1979.

Hoeffer, B. Children's acquisition of sex-role behavior in lesbian mother families. *Journal of American Orthopsychiatry,* 1981, *Vol. 51,* No. 3, 536-545.

Kirkpatrick, M., Smith, K., & Roy, R. Lesbian mothers and their children: a comparative study. *Journal of American Orthopsychiatry,* 1981, *Vol. 51,* No. 3, 545-552.

Lewin, E. Lesbianism and motherhoood: implications for child custody. *Human Organization,* 1981, *Vol. 40,* No. 1.

Lewin, E., & Lyons, T. Everything in its place: the coexistence of lesbianism and motherhood. In W. Paul *et al.* (Eds.), *Homosexuality.* Beverly Hills: Sage Publications, 1982.

Mandel, J., Hotvedt, M., & Green, R. The lesbian parent: comparison of heterosexual and homosexual mothers and children. Paper presented at meetings of the American Psychological Association, New York, 1979.

Martin, D., & Lyon, P. Lesbian/woman. New York: Bantam, 1972.

Rivera, R. Our straight-laced judges: the legal position of homosexual persons in America. *The Hastings Law Journal,* March 1979, *Vol. 30.*